Comparative Effectiveness Review
Number 140

Chronic Urinary Retention: Comparative Effectiveness and Harms of Treatments

Prepared for:
Agency for Healthcare Research and Quality
U.S. Department of Health and Human Services
540 Gaither Road
Rockville, MD 20850
www.ahrq.gov

Contract No. 290-2007-10064-I

Prepared by:
Minnesota Evidence-based Practice Center
Minneapolis, MN

Investigators:
Michelle Brasure, Ph.D., M.S.P.H., M.L.I.S.
Howard A. Fink, M.D., M.P.H.
Michael Risk, M.D.
Roderick MacDonald, M.S.
Tatyana Shamliyan, M.D.
Jeannine Ouellette
Dongjuan Xu, M.Sc.
Mary Butler, Ph.D.
Robert L. Kane, M.D.
Timothy J. Wilt, M.D., M.P.H.

AHRQ Publication No. 14-EHC041-EF
September 2014

This report is based on research conducted by the Minnesota Evidence-based Practice Center (EPC) under contract to the Agency for Healthcare Research and Quality (AHRQ), Rockville, MD (Contract No. 290-2007-10064-I). The findings and conclusions in this document are those of the authors, who are responsible for its contents; the findings and conclusions do not necessarily represent the views of AHRQ. Therefore, no statement in this report should be construed as an official position of AHRQ or of the U.S. Department of Health and Human Services.

The information in this report is intended to help health care decisionmakers—patients and clinicians, health system leaders, and policymakers, among others—make well informed decisions and thereby improve the quality of health care services. This report is not intended to be a substitute for the application of clinical judgment. Anyone who makes decisions concerning the provision of clinical care should consider this report in the same way as any medical reference and in conjunction with all other pertinent information, i.e., in the context of available resources and circumstances presented by individual patients.

This report may be used, in whole or in part, as the basis for development of clinical practice guidelines and other quality enhancement tools, or as a basis for reimbursement and coverage policies. AHRQ or U.S. Department of Health and Human Services endorsement of such derivative products may not be stated or implied.

This report may periodically be assessed for the urgency to update. If an assessment is done, the resulting surveillance report describing the methodology and findings will be found on the Effective Health Care Program Web site at www.effectivehealthcare.ahrq.gov. Search on the title of the report.

This document is in the public domain and may be used and reprinted without special permission. Citation of the source is appreciated.

Persons using assistive technology may not be able to fully access information in this report. For assistance contact EffectiveHealthCare@ahrq.hhs.gov.

None of the investigators have any affiliations or financial involvement that conflicts with the material presented in this report.

Suggested citation: Brasure M, Fink HA, Risk M, MacDonald R, Shamliyan T, Ouellette J, Xu D, Butler M, Kane RL, Wilt TJ. Chronic Urinary Retention: Comparative Effectiveness and Harms of Treatments. Comparative Effectiveness Review No. 140. (Prepared by the Minnesota Evidence-based Practice Center under Contract No. 290-2007-10064-I.) AHRQ Publication No. 14-EHC041-EF. Rockville, MD: Agency for Healthcare Research and Quality; September 2014. www.effectivehealthcare.ahrq.gov/reports/final.cfm.

Preface

The Agency for Healthcare Research and Quality (AHRQ), through its Evidence-based Practice Centers (EPCs), sponsors the development of systematic reviews to assist public- and private-sector organizations in their efforts to improve the quality of health care in the United States. These reviews provide comprehensive, science-based information on common, costly medical conditions and new health care technologies and strategies.

Systematic reviews are the building blocks underlying evidence-based practice; they focus attention on the strength and limits of evidence from research studies about the effectiveness and safety of a clinical intervention. In the context of developing recommendations for practice, systematic reviews can help clarify whether assertions about the value of the intervention are based on strong evidence from clinical studies. For more information about AHRQ EPC systematic reviews, see www.effectivehealthcare.ahrq.gov/reference/purpose.cfm.

AHRQ expects that these systematic reviews will be helpful to health plans, providers, purchasers, government programs, and the health care system as a whole. Transparency and stakeholder input are essential to the Effective Health Care Program. Please visit the Web site (www.effectivehealthcare.ahrq.gov) to see draft research questions and reports or to join an email list to learn about new program products and opportunities for input.

We welcome comments on this systematic review. They may be sent by mail to the Task Order Officer named below at: Agency for Healthcare Research and Quality, 540 Gaither Road, Rockville, MD 20850, or by email to epc@ahrq.hhs.gov.

Richard G. Kronick, Ph.D.
Director, Agency for Healthcare Research
and Quality

Yen-pin Chiang, Ph.D.
Acting Deputy Director, Center for
Evidence and Practice Improvement
Agency for Healthcare Research and Quality

Stephanie Chang, M.D., M.P.H.
Director, EPC Program
Center for Evidence
and Practice Improvement
Agency for Healthcare Research and Quality

Suchitra Iyer, Ph.D.
Task Order Officer
Center for Evidence and Practice
Improvement
Agency for Healthcare Research and Quality

Acknowledgments

We would like to thank Marilyn Eells for outstanding editing support.

Key Informants

In designing the study questions, the EPC consulted a panel of Key Informants who represent subject experts and end-users of research. Key Informant input can inform key issues related to the topic of the technical brief. Key Informants are not involved in the analysis of the evidence or the writing of the report. Therefore, in the end, study questions, design, methodological approaches, and/or conclusions do not necessarily represent the views of individual Key Informants.

Key Informants must disclose any financial conflicts of interest greater than $10,000 and any other relevant business or professional conflicts of interest. Because of their role as end-users, individuals with potential conflicts may be retained. The TOO and the EPC work to balance, manage, or mitigate any conflicts of interest.

The list of Key Informants who participated in developing this report follows:

Victor Nitti, M.D.
New York University
New York, NY

Vivian W. Sung, M.D., M.P.H.
Women and Infants' Hospital of Rhode Island
Providence, RI

John Wei, M.D., M.S.
University of Michigan
Ann Arbor, MI

Technical Expert Panel

In designing the study questions and methodology at the outset of this report, the EPC consulted several technical and content experts. Broad expertise and perspectives were sought. Divergent and conflicted opinions are common and perceived as healthy scientific discourse that results in a thoughtful, relevant systematic review. Therefore, in the end, study questions, design, methodologic approaches, and/or conclusions do not necessarily represent the views of individual technical and content experts.

Technical Experts must disclose any financial conflicts of interest greater than $10,000 and any other relevant business or professional conflicts of interest. Because of their unique clinical or content expertise, individuals with potential conflicts may be retained. The TOO and the EPC work to balance, manage, or mitigate any potential conflicts of interest identified.

The list of Technical Experts who participated in developing this report follows:

Amy Driscoll, B.S.N, C.U.R.N., C.C.C.N.
Minneapolis VA Health Care System
Minneapolis, MN

Mary Ann Forciea, M.D.
University of Pennsylvania
Philadelphia, PA

Gary Goldish, M.D.
Minneapolis VA Health Care System
Minneapolis, MN

Patricia Lapera, M.P.H., C.H.E.S.
American Urological Association
Linthicum, MD

Vivian W. Sung, M.D., M.P.H.
Women and Infants' Hospital of Rhode Island
Providence, RI

John Wei, M.D., M.S.
University of Michigan
Ann Arbor, MI

Peer Reviewers

Prior to publication of the final evidence report, EPCs sought input from independent Peer Reviewers without financial conflicts of interest. However, the conclusions and synthesis of the scientific literature presented in this report does not necessarily represent the views of individual reviewers.

Peer Reviewers must disclose any financial conflicts of interest greater than $10,000 and any other relevant business or professional conflicts of interest. Because of their unique clinical or content expertise, individuals with potential nonfinancial conflicts may be retained. The TOO and the EPC work to balance, manage, or mitigate any potential nonfinancial conflicts of interest identified.

The list of Peer Reviewers follows:

James Quentin Clemens, M.D
University of Michigan
Ann Arbor, MI

Ananias Diokno, M.D.
Oakland University William Beaumont School of Medicine
Rochester, MI

Carlo Negro, M.D., FEBU
Ospedale Cardinal Massaia - ASL AT
AT Torino, Italy

Brian Selius, D.O.
Northeast Ohio Medical University
Youngstown, OH

Chronic Urinary Retention: Comparative Effectiveness and Harms of Treatments

Structured Abstract

Objective. To determine the effectiveness and comparative effectiveness of treatments for chronic urinary retention (CUR), also termed partial or persistent urinary retention or incomplete bladder emptying, in adults.

Data sources. Ovid MEDLINE® and the Cochrane Central Register of Controlled Trials bibliographic databases; hand searches of references of relevant studies.

Review methods. Two investigators screened abstracts and full-text articles of identified references for eligibility. Eligible studies included randomized controlled trials and prospective cohort studies enrolling patients with CUR. Primary outcomes included rate of urinary tract infections, urinary symptom or quality-of-life score category, and successful trial without catheter. Intermediate outcomes included postvoid residual (PVR) urine volume and continuous measures of urinary symptoms or quality of life. We extracted data, assessed risk of bias on individual studies, and evaluated strength of evidence for each comparison and outcome.

Results. We identified 11 publications reporting original research and 2 relevant systematic reviews that met eligibility criteria. Results are analyzed by etiology: obstructive, nonobstructive, and mixed populations/unknown causes. Only three studies addressed obstructive causes of CUR; all studied men with bladder outlet obstruction due to benign prostatic enlargement. Low-strength evidence suggested that transurethral resection of the prostate and microwave therapy achieved similar improvements in the rates of successful trial without catheter at 6 months posttreatment. Evidence was insufficient to draw conclusions regarding other outcomes because estimates were imprecise, risk of bias was moderate, and consistency could not be evaluated. Evidence for other treatment comparisons for CUR from obstructive causes was insufficient to conclude that one treatment was more effective than the comparison. Four small studies and one systematic review assessed treatments for CUR from nonobstructive causes. A previous systematic review provided low-strength evidence that neuromodulation improves the rate at which patients with Fowler's syndrome can be catheter free after treatment. Low-strength evidence suggested that botulinum toxin injected into the urethral sphincter may not improve PVR volumes. Two studies and one systematic review addressed CUR treatments in mixed populations or CUR from unknown causes. Evidence from original research was insufficient to conclude that one treatment was any more or less effective than another. Evidence on harms was inconsistently reported across all interventions, and no differences were detected across treatment groups; however, studies were not adequately powered to detect differences in harms across groups.

Conclusions. We identified few studies; most were small and had methodological flaws. Evidence was insufficient due to risk of bias and imprecision, and we were not able to evaluate consistency of results across studies. Further research should address conceptual issues in studying CUR as well as strengthening the evidence base with adequately powered controlled trials or prospective cohort studies for populations and interventions common in practice.

Contents

Introduction 1
    Background 1
Methods 3
Results 5
    Search Results 5
    Comparative Effectiveness of Treatments for CUR: Obstructive Causes 6
        Benefits 6
        Harms 6
    Comparative Effectiveness of Treatments for CUR: Non-Obstructive Causes 8
        Benefits 8
        Harms 8
    Comparative Effectiveness of Treatments for CUR: Mixed Populations/Unknown Causes .. 10
        Benefits 10
        Harms 10
Discussion 12
    Applicability 12
    Limitations 12
    Future Research Needs 13
Conclusions 14
References 15
Abbreviations 17

Tables
Table 1. PICOTS framework 2
Table 2. Summary outcomes and strength of evidence: treatments for obstructive chronic
        urinary retention 7
Table 3. Description and conclusions from previous systematic review relevant to treatment
        for CUR from non-obstructive causes 8
Table 4. Summary outcomes, adverse events, and strength of evidence assessments of
        treatments for CUR from non-obstructive causes 9
Table 5. Description and conclusions from previous systematic reviews of treatments for
        CUR in mixed populations or unknown causes 10
Table 6. Summary outcomes, adverse events, and strength of evidence of treatments for
        CUR in mixed populations or unknown causes 11

Figures
Figure 1. Literature flow diagram 5

Appendixes
Appendix A. CUR Treatments
Appendix B. Analytical Framework
Appendix C. Search Strategy
Appendix D. Inclusion Criteria
Appendix E. Excluded Studies
Appendix F. Description and Characteristics of Included Studies
Appendix G. Risk of Bias and Quality

Appendix H. Detailed Results
Appendix I. Strength of Evidence
Appendix J. Ongoing Studies
Appendix K. Future Research Needs

Introduction

Background

Persistent partial retention of urine or chronic urinary retention (CUR) is a common problem for which we have little understanding in terms of prevalence, natural history, prognosis, or efficacy and comparative effectiveness of treatments. Also unclear are whether and when to suspect, screen, or treat patients for CUR. Standard diagnostic criteria (including the duration and volume of post-void residual [PVR] urine necessary for a diagnosis) have not been established for chronic urinary retention.[1,2] Researchers often define CUR as PVR urine volume greater than 300 ml; however, some studies define it as 100 ml, 400 ml, or 500 ml.[1]

CUR may be either asymptomatic or associated with lower urinary tract symptoms such as urinary frequency, urgency, or incontinence.[3] Elevated PVR or CUR can increase risk for urinary tract infections (UTI) and renal failure.[3] Some studies of men with lower urinary tract symptoms and CUR indicate increased risk of acute urinary retention (AUR), renal failure, and lower likelihood that benign prostatic hypertrophy surgery will improve urinary symptoms.[2] A threshold PVR urine volume associated with these consequences is unclear, although negative outcomes have been demonstrated in men with PVR volumes over 500 ml.[1] We do not know if these findings are applicable to asymptomatic CUR.

CUR is almost always caused by another (often concomitant) medical condition. Causes of CUR are commonly categorized as obstructive or non-obstructive. In men, the most prevalent obstructive cause is bladder outlet obstruction associated with benign prostatic enlargement. As many as 25 percent of men who undergo prostate surgery for benign prostatic enlargement have CUR.[2] Obstructive causes of CUR in women include complications from surgery for stress urinary incontinence and pelvic organ prolapse. In both sexes, urethral strictures and pelvic masses are obstructive causes.[3] CUR not caused by obstruction is typically due to detrusor underactivity, which can be neurogenic (damage to nerves that innervate the bladder in conditions such as multiple sclerosis, spinal cord injury) or myogenic (damage to the smooth muscle of the bladder).[1,4] An additional non-obstructive cause of CUR is Fowler's syndrome, which affects mainly young women, is characterized by urinary retention due to a failure of urethral sphincter relaxation,[5] and is not well recognized in the United States.

The goal treatment is to improve function and/or quality of life and reduce complications to an extent meaningful to patients. Treatment and management options (Appendix A) depend on etiology. Most approaches (including surgery, minimally invasive procedures, and drugs) address the underlying condition or mechanical cause (e.g., benign prostatic enlargement, neurogenic bladder) rather than specifically addressing CUR. When treatment fails to alleviate CUR, catheterization can be used for bladder management. Harms are specific to the interventions and may include infection and surgical complications. Our review addresses the following Key Questions:

Key Question 1: What are the effectiveness and comparative effectiveness of treatments for chronic urinary retention in adults?
   a. With male-specific etiologies?
   b. With female-specific etiologies?
   c. With non sex-specific etiologies

d. What patient or condition characteristics (e.g., age, severity, etc.) modify the effectiveness of treatment?

Key Question 2: What are the harms and comparative harms of treatments for chronic urinary retention in adults?
   a. With male-specific etiologies?
   b. With female-specific etiologies?
   c. With non sex-specific etiologies?
   d. What patient or condition characteristics (e.g., age, severity, etc.) modify the harms of treatment?

The PICOTS (Population, Intervention, Comparison, Outcomes, Timing, and Setting) addressed by our Key Questions are described in Table 1. An analytical framework describing the relationship between the PICOTS elements appears in Appendix B.

Table 1. PICOTS framework

PICOTS Element	Inclusion Criteria
Population	Adults 18 or older with CUR (a persistently elevated PVR volume of 100 ml or greater). Patients with acute or transient retention attributed to drug side effects, medical or surgical procedures, or infection/inflammation were excluded.
Intervention	Catheterization Surgical interventions (etiology-specific): prostate surgery (BPH), corrections for incontinence surgery (surgical complication to incontinence surgery, pelvic organ prolapse repair (pelvic organ prolapse), sacral nerve stimulation (neurologic), pessary placement. Pharmacologic treatments: alpha blockers (AB), 5-alpha reductase inhibitors (5-ARI), AB + 5-ARI combination treatment available in the United States Urinary diversion
Comparator	Placebo or any of above interventions
Outcomes	Primary outcomes: AUR; UTI; TWOC; categorical change in urinary symptom or quality of life scale scores. Adverse effects: any reported (e.g., death, surgical complications, bleeding, urinary incontinence)
Timing	Any treatment duration
Setting	Any treatment setting

Abbreviations: AUR = acute urinary retention; BPH = benign prostatic hypertrophy; CUR = chronic urinary retention; PICOTS = population, intervention, comparator, outcomes, timing, and setting; PVR = postvoid residual; TWOC = trial without catheterization, UTI = urinary tract infection

Methods

The draft Key Questions developed during AHRQ's Topic Refinement process were posted for public comment from October 22, 2012, through November 19, 2012. The comments received suggested that changes to the scope of the draft Key Questions were unnecessary. Comments did, however, suggest that we call the condition "incomplete bladder emptying" or "elevated postvoid residual" instead of CUR. We addressed these comments and conducted preliminary literature reviews in developing the draft protocol during the Comparative Effectiveness Review phase of the project. We next convened a Technical Expert Panel (TEP) of clinicians and researchers in urology, primary care, physical medicine and rehabilitation, and gynecology for topical guidance during the CER. We solicited their expertise in defining populations, interventions, comparisons, and outcomes, and in identifying particular studies. The Key Informants and members of the TEP were required to disclose any financial conflicts of interest greater than $10,000 and any other relevant business or professional conflicts. Any potential conflicts of interest were balanced or mitigated. TEP members did not perform analysis of any kind, nor did they contribute to the writing of this report. Members of the TEP were invited to provide feedback on an initial draft of the review protocol. That draft was then revised, reviewed by AHRQ, and posted for public access on the AHRQ Effective Health Care Program Web site.

We registered the protocol for this review with the International Prospective Registry of Systematic Reviews, PROSPERO (registration number: CRD42013004639). The final version is available at effectivehealthcare.ahrq.gov/index.cfm/search-for-guides-reviews-and-reports/?productid=1539&pageaction=displayproduct. We conducted bibliographic database searches in MEDLINE and the Cochrane Central Register of Controlled Trials (CENTRAL) to identify previous systematic reviews, randomized controlled trials, and prospective cohort studies published from 1946 through February 15, 2014. Because the natural history of CUR is poorly understood, controlled studies are especially important; without a control group, we could not know whether changes in CUR outcomes were due to interventions or part of the natural history of the condition. We searched only for the CUR concept and used relevant medical subject headings and natural language terms to identify studies (Appendix C). We narrowed the search by using filters designed to select experimental designs.[6] Bibliographic database searches were supplemented with backward citation searches of highly relevant systematic reviews. Two investigators reviewed titles and abstracts to identify those potentially meeting inclusion criteria (Appendix D). All controlled studies that addressed the PICOTS described previously were eligible and included. Two investigators worked independently to screen the full text of studies identified as potentially meeting inclusion criteria. Differences in inclusion decisions were addressed through consultation; a third investigator was consulted when necessary.

We first assessed the relevance of systematic reviews that met inclusion criteria. If we determined that certain Key Questions or comparisons addressed in the previous systematic review were relevant to our review, we assessed the quality of the methodology using modified AMSTAR criteria.[7] When prior systematic reviews were assessed as sufficient quality, and when the review assessed strength of evidence or provided sufficient information for it to be assessed, we used the conclusions from that review to replace the de novo process. If additional studies on these comparisons were identified, we updated the systematic review results. We then abstracted data from eligible trials and prospective cohort studies not included in previous systematic reviews that addressed comparisons not sufficiently addressed by a previous eligible systematic review. One investigator abstracted the relevant data into the Systematic Review Data

Repository tool and/or directly to evidence tables. A second investigator reviewed evidence tables and verified them for accuracy. Based on judgments of selection bias, performance and detection bias (allocation concealment and blinding), attrition bias, reporting bias, and other sources of bias, investigators assessed overall risk of bias for each eligible study.

We categorized eligible studies into groups for analysis based on similar populations. We conducted a qualitative synthesis because of heterogeneity in populations, interventions, and outcomes studied.

We evaluated overall strength of evidence for primary outcomes for each treatment comparison and outcome. We included the following primary outcomes a priori: rates of AUR, UTI, successful trial without catheter, and categorical measures of urinary symptom or quality of life scales. We treated change in PVR urine volume and continuous measures of urinary symptoms and/or quality of life as intermediate outcomes. We specifically analyzed PVR to assess whether patients no longer met CUR diagnostic criteria and to better understand the impact of treatment on urinary symptoms and PVR. We abstracted data on any harms reported. Given the relative infrequency of harms occurrence and the inconsistency in reporting harms across studies, we did not formally assess strength of evidence for all harms and focused instead on intervention benefits. In some cases, events we categorized as primary outcomes are also considered treatment harms. For instance, UTI is thought to be both a consequence of CUR; as well as a harm associated with many of the interventions. We chose to categorize this variable as a primary outcome instead of a harm. As a primary outcome, rate of UTI captures the net amount of UTI prevented rather than caused by the intervention. Similarly, we categorized surgical intervention, considered a harm of some CUR interventions, as a primary outcome. Our assessment of strength of evidence for these outcomes is discussed in the benefits section.

Strength of evidence assessments (high, moderate, low, or insufficient) were based on four required domains: (1) study limitations (internal validity); (2) directness (single, direct link between intervention and outcome); (3) consistency (similarity of effect direction and size); and (4) precision (degree of certainty around an estimate).[8] A low strength of evidence required at least moderate or low risk of bias and precision. Moderate or high strength of evidence assessments required directness and/or consistency as well. Evidence was rated insufficient if outcomes differences between groups were not significant and imprecise.

We evaluated the applicability or generalizability of study results according to the PICOTS framework, paying particular attention to narrow eligibility criteria and patient characteristics that may differ from those of individuals in the community undergoing treatment for CUR from similar causes.[9]

Results

Search Results

Our search identified 1,521 citations, of which 38 required full-text review after title and abstract screening (Figure 1). Of the 38 full text articles screened, we identified 11 eligible studies representing 11 unique reports of original research[10-20] and two relevant systematic reviews.[21, 22] Studies excluded after full-text review are listed in Appendix E along with exclusion reasons.

Figure 1. Literature flow diagram

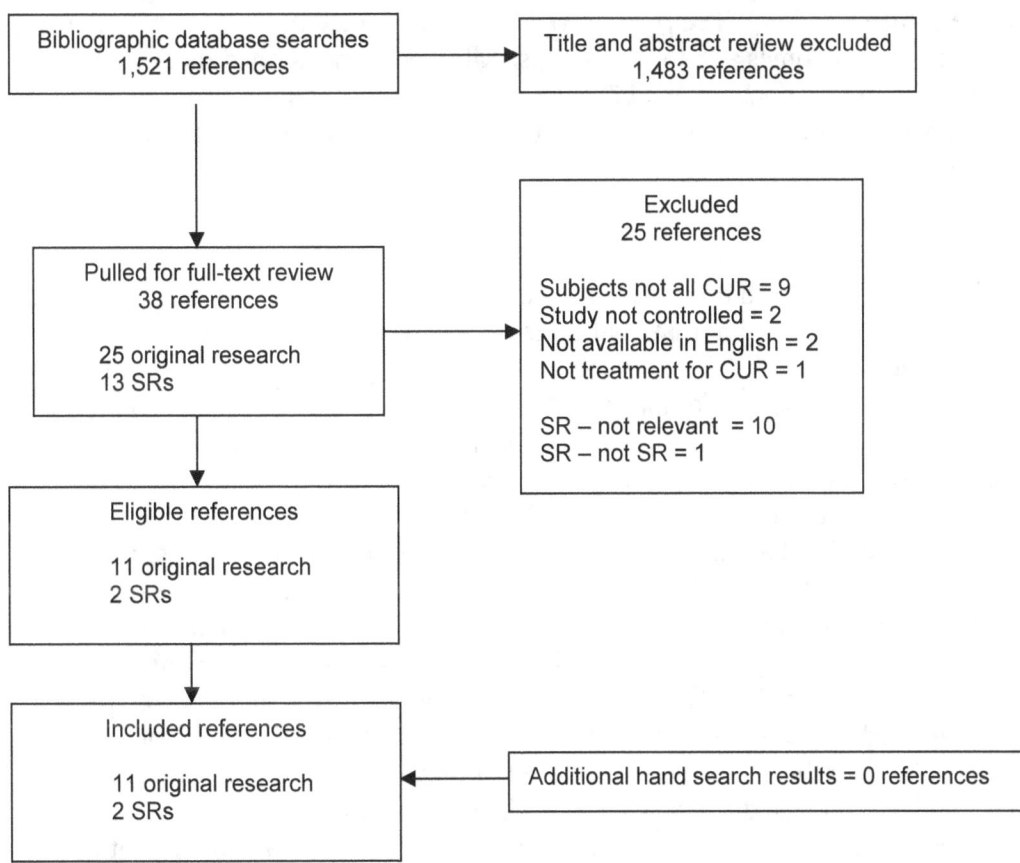

We categorized studies into groups for synthesis based on CUR etiology:
- CUR from obstructive causes
- CUR from non-obstructive causes
- CUR in mixed populations/unknown causes

Eligible studies rarely specified CUR duration. We included any study that treated CUR related to chronic conditions or that specified persistent or multiple measurements. The appendices of this report provide detailed information about the included studies: characteristics of the individual studies (Appendix F); risk of bias and quality assessments of original research and systematic reviews (Appendix G); summaries of included studies, analysis, and detailed outcomes tables (Appendix H); and detailed strength of evidence assessments (Appendix I).

Comparative Effectiveness of Treatments for CUR: Obstructive Causes

We identified three eligible studies for treatment of CUR from obstructive causes; all three were RCTs that compared treatments for CUR in men with bladder outlet obstruction due to benign prostatic enlargement.[12, 13, 19] All defined CUR as persistent PVR >300ml. Participants also had to have other lower urinary tract symptoms. The mean age of the 243 men enrolled was 71 years. Two studies reported mean baseline International Prostate Symptom Scores (IPSS) and PVR volumes with a mean baseline total IPSS of 21.4 (indicating severe symptoms) and mean baseline PVR volume of 626 ml. All three trials compared surgery (transurethral resection of the prostate [TURP] or prostate enucleation) to a less invasive intervention (laser, microwave, clean intermittent sterile catheterization [CISC]). Two trials were conducted in Europe and one in Asia. All trials measured outcomes at 6 to 7.5 months. All three demonstrated methodological problems (i.e., inability to blind patient and provider, allocation concealment) and each was assessed as having overall moderate risk of bias. Table 2 provides a summary of primary outcomes and adverse effects.

Benefits

Two of the three RCTs reported on five primary outcomes (UTI, treatment failure, TWOC, need for surgical intervention, and International Prostate Symptom Score (IPSS) category).[12, 19] The third RCT assessed only intermediate outcomes, analysis of which is not included here.[13] Schelin et al., reported that 33 percent of the microwave therapy group and 22 percent of the TURP group experienced a UTI (diagnostic criteria not specified); 79 percent of the microwave therapy group and 88 percent of the TURP group were catheter free at 6 months; 7 percent of the microwave therapy group and 4 percent of the TURP group maintained PVR volumes above 300 ml.[12] Neither trial self-identified as testing for equivalence or noninferiority. Low-strength evidence suggested that the rates at which men were catheter free at 6 months were similar between TURP and microwave therapy. Data was not available to prespecify a minimum important difference in the group proportions for this population-treatment-outcome, but equivalence could be inferred at any MID at or above a 25 percent differential ($\alpha=.05$; $\beta=.80$).

Gujral, et al., reported that 5 percent of TURP and 3 percent of laser therapy groups had experienced UTIs at 7.5 months.[19] No one in the TURP group and three in the laser group required surgery. Neither of these differences was statistically significant.

The third trial compared TURP to clean intermittent self-catheterization but did not evaluate any of our primary outcomes.[13]

All treatments tested in the three trials reduced PVR volumes, and the trials reported no statistically significant differences between comparisons.

Harms

Each study measured adverse effects differently, reporting either incidence of specific adverse effects, incidence of serious adverse effects, or postsurgical complication rates. Reported harms included death, septicemia, bleeding, blood transfusions, and surgical complications. Harms did not differ between surgery versus microwave therapy or between surgery (TURP or prostate enucleation) versus clean intermittent self-catheterization, but a larger proportion of patients in the TURP group experienced complications (death, septicemia, bleeding, blood transfusions, and surgical complications) than in the laser group.[19]

Table 2. Summary outcomes and strength of evidence: treatments for obstructive chronic urinary retention

Study (n); Comparison; Inclusion Criteria; Design	Outcomes	Results	Strength of Evidence (Explanation for Assessment)
Schelin 2006[12] (n=120) TURP or prostate enucleation surgery vs. microwave therapy Men ≥45 years of age with symptomatic BPH and PVR >300mL RCT	**Primary outcomes** Urinary tract infection	NS RR 1.49 [0.82 to 2.71]	Insufficient (moderate risk of bias, imprecise, unclear consistency)
	TWOC	NS RR 0.89 [0.76 to 1.05]	Low (moderate risk of bias, unclear consistency)
	Adverse effects Serious adverse events	NS	NA
Ghalayini 2005[13] (n=51) TURP vs. CISC Men with LUTS, baseline IPSS >7 and PVR >300 mL RCT	**Primary outcomes** None reported	NR	Insufficient (no data)
	Adverse effects Complication rate	NS	NA
Gujral 2000[19] (n=82) TURP vs. laser therapy Men with LUTS and baseline IPSS ≥8 and PVR >300mL RCT	**Primary outcomes** Urinary tract infection	NS RR 1.73 [0.16 to 18.31]	Insufficient (moderate risk of bias, imprecise, unclear consistency)
	Surgical intervention	NS RR 0.12 [0.01 to 2.32]	Insufficient (moderate risk of bias, imprecise, unclear consistency)
	IPSS Category (Good, Fair, Poor)	NS RR 1.27 [95% CI 0.97 to 1.68]	Insufficient (high risk of bias, unclear consistency)
	IPSS Category (Good, Fair, Poor) adjusted**	TURP ↑ RR 3.9 [95% CI 1.0 to 14.3]	Low (moderate risk of bias, unclear consistency)
	Adverse effects Complication rate	TURP ↑	NA

BPH = benign prostatic hyperplasia; CI= confidence intervals; CISC = clean intermittent self-catheterization; IPSS = International Prostate Symptom Score (range 0 [mild symptoms] to 35 [severe symptoms]); LUTS = lower urinary tract symptoms; MD = mean difference; NA = not assessed; NR = not reported; NS = no statistically significant difference; PVR = post void residual; QoL = quality of life; RCT = randomized controlled trial; RR = risk ratio; TURP = transurethral resection of the prostate; TWOC = trial without catheter

** Adjustment for differences between groups at baseline in marital status and prostate volume

Comparative Effectiveness of Treatments for CUR: Non-Obstructive Causes

Four small efficacy studies and one systematic review compared treatments for CUR attributed to non-obstructive causes in adults. The systematic review, conducted by the Cochrane Incontinence Group, was assessed as having good quality.[21] Herbison et al. reviewed sacral neuromodulation with implanted devices for urinary storage and voiding dysfunction in adults.[21] We report the conclusion from that review in lieu of de novo abstraction and analysis of the original research (Table 3).[17,18,20]

Original research included three RCTs with moderate risk of bias and one prospective cohort design. Studies enrolled a total of 139 patients with sample sizes ranging from 13 to 86. The mean age of enrolled patients was 54, with a range from 46 to 66. Fifty-one percent of subjects were men. Baseline mean IPSS score was 21.4 across the two studies that measured IPSS, suggesting a severe level of symptoms. Neurogenic disorders among the patients included multiple sclerosis (64 percent), spinal cord injury (7 percent), and other conditions such as stroke or traumatic brain injury (29 percent). In the three studies reporting condition duration, patients had been living with these neurogenic disorders for an average of 13 years. Trials were conducted in Europe and Asia. Three studies compared botulinum A injected into the urethral sphincter to an inactive control (placebo, lidocaine, usual care). The fourth study compared bethanechol/prostaglandin (BC/PGE2) to placebo.

Benefits

Herbison et al. addressed one comparison relevant to our review—early (immediate) implant versus a delayed implant (waitlist) in treating CUR from non-obstructive retention.[21] Low-strength evidence suggests that early sacral neuromodulation with implanted devices is effective in achieving catheter-free status and reducing PVR in patients with idiopathic non-obstructive CUR. Remaining evidence was insufficient due to indirect outcomes and imprecise estimates created by the wide confidence intervals of underpowered studies (Table 4).

Harms

None of these studies found differences in the rates of serious or any adverse effects between treatment groups, though studies were not adequately powered to detect these.

Table 3. Description and conclusions from previous systematic review relevant to treatment for CUR from non-obstructive causes

Study Information	Literature Through; SR Quality	Population; Relevant Comparison	Results; Conclusion Strength of Evidence
Herbison 2009[21] (Cochrane Incontinence Group) Sacral neuromodulation with implanted devices for urinary storage and voiding dysfunction in adults 1 RCT	Literature search through February, 2009 Good	Patients with complete or partial idiopathic urinary retention Immediate/delayed implant (1 trial with CUR patients)	Catheter free: Early>Delay PVR: Early>Delay Low

RCT = randomized controlled trial; PVR = post void residual; SR = systematic review; UTI = urinary tract infection

Table 4. Summary outcomes, adverse events, and strength of evidence assessments of treatments for CUR from non-obstructive causes

Study (n); Comparison; Inclusion Criteria; Design	Outcomes	Results	Strength of Evidence
Gallien 2005[14] (n=86) Botulinum A toxin vs. Placebo MS patients with DSD. Patients with CUR had PVR of 100 to 500 ml RCT	**Primary outcomes** Urinary tract infection **Adverse effects** Serious adverse events	NS RR 1.21 [95% CI 0.66 to 2.25] NS	Insufficient (moderate risk of bias, indirect, imprecise, unclear consistency) NA
Hindley 2004[15] (n=19) Bethanechol chloride plus prostaglandin E2 vs. placebo Patients with suspected detrusor under-activity, defined as PVR >300 mL in the absence of BPO RCT	**Primary outcomes** TWOC **Adverse effects** Any adverse events	NS NS	Insufficient (moderate risk of bias, indirect, imprecise, unclear consistency) NA
de Sèze 2002[17] (n=13) Botulinum A toxin vs. Lidocaine Patients with DSD. CUR defined as PVR >100 ml RCT	**Primary outcomes:** None reported **Adverse effects:** Any adverse events	NR NS	Insufficient (no data) NA
Chen 2004[16] (n=21) Botulinum A toxin vs. usual care Patients with urethral sphincter pseudo-dyssynergia due to chronic cerebrovascular accidents or intracranial lesions Prospective cohort study	**Primary outcomes:** None reported **Adverse effects:** Serious adverse events	NR NS	Insufficient (no data) NA

BPO = Benign Prostatic Obstruction; CI = confidence intervals; DSD = detrusor sphincter dyssynergia; IPSS = International Prostate Symptom Score (range 0 [mild symptoms] to 35 [severe symptoms]); MD = mean difference; MS = multiple sclerosis; NA = not assessed; NR = not reported; NS = no statistically significant difference; PVR = post void residual ; QoL = quality of life; RCT = randomized controlled trial; RR = risk ratio; TWOC = trial without catheter

Comparative Effectiveness of Treatments for CUR: Mixed Populations/Unknown Causes

Four studies (original research) and one systematic review addressed six different comparisons for treatments for CUR in mixed populations or CUR from unknown causes. One comparison was adequately addressed by a previous systematic review.[21, 22] The systematic review was conducted by the Cochrane Incontinence Group and assessed as being of good quality. We report conclusions from that review in lieu of de novo abstraction and analysis of the original research (Table 5).[18, 20]

Benefits

Moore et al. compared clean versus sterile catheterization technique.[22] They found data from three studies insufficient to draw conclusions. Only one of these trials had CUR as an enrollment criterion and was eligible for our review.[20] Because the results from the three trials eligible for the Cochrane review were consistent and the data were assessed as insufficient, we reiterate their conclusion of insufficient evidence for this comparison.

Two small RCTs studied efficacy and comparative effectiveness of CUR interventions in populations with CUR from mixed obstructive and non-obstructive or unknown causes (Table 6). In one study of 19 women with obstructed voiding or retention associated with Fowler's syndrome, evidence for treating CUR with sildenafil was insufficient to draw conclusions about effectiveness. The other RCT evaluated intermittent versus indwelling catheterization among elderly women with CUR admitted to a geriatric rehabilitation ward. This study provided insufficient information to draw conclusions about the rates of UTI with intermittent versus indwelling catheterization but provided low-strength evidence of no difference between the proportion of patients able to go without catheter after intermittent or indwelling catheter treatment. However, we could not determine whether these patients were truly CUR patients and not suffering from transient urinary retention.

Harms

Adverse effects were measured differently in each RCT. These events were rare, and results did not differ between treatment groups, though studies were not adequately powered to detect such differences.

Table 5. Description and conclusions from previous systematic reviews of treatments for CUR in mixed populations or unknown causes

Study Information	Literature Through; SR Quality	Population; Relevant Comparison	Results; Conclusion Strength of Evidence
Moore 2009 [22] (Cochrane Incontinence Group) Long-term bladder management by intermittent catheterization in adults and children 3 RCTs	Literature search through June 2007 Good	Adults and children with incomplete bladder emptying Sterile technique/clean technique (3 trials; only one with only CUR population)	The evidence was insufficient to permit a conclusion for rates of UTI

PVR = post void residual; SR=systematic review; UTI = urinary tract infection

Table 6. Summary outcomes, adverse events, and strength of evidence of treatments for CUR in mixed populations or unknown causes

Study (n); Comparison; Inclusion Criteria; Design	Outcomes	Result	Strength of Evidence
Datta 2007[10] (n=19) Sildenafil vs. Placebo Women with obstructed voiding or retention associated with Fowler's Syndrome RCT	**Primary outcomes** Urinary tract infection **Adverse effects** Death Clinical deterioration (Total not reported)	NS NS	Insufficient (moderate risk of bias, imprecise, unclear consistency) NA
Tang 2006[11] (n=81) Intermittent urinary catheterization vs. indwelling urinary catheterization Elderly women admitted to a female geriatric rehabilitation ward. Patients with a PVR >150 ml were regarded as having urinary retention. If PVR remained ≥300 ml, the subjects were then randomized RCT	**Primary outcomes** Urinary tract infection TWOC **Adverse effects** Total adverse effects	NS NS RR 0.86 [95% CI 0.59 to 1.25] NS	Insufficient (moderate risk of bias, imprecise, unclear consistency) Low (moderate risk of bias, unclear consistency) NA

CI = confidence interval; NA = not assessed; NR = not reported; NS = no statistically significant difference; PVR = post void residual; RCT = randomized controlled trial; RR = risk ratio; TWOC = trial without catheter

Discussion

Overall, we identified few studies that enrolled patients with CUR. Those that did typically enrolled adults with CUR as well as the contributing condition (e.g., benign prostatic enlargement or multiple sclerosis). Eligible studies were generally small and had moderate risk of bias. We grouped similar populations for analysis. We found that many of the possible CUR etiologies had not been studied in controlled trials. For etiologies that were studied, evidence was most often insufficient to draw conclusions about efficacy and comparative effectiveness of various interventions.

We identified only three studies that examined the treatment for CUR from obstructive causes. All addressed CUR associated with bladder outlet obstruction from benign prostatic enlargement and enrolled men with CUR and urinary symptoms.

- Data were insufficient to draw conclusions regarding most outcomes for each comparison. Low-strength evidence suggested no statistical difference between TURP and microwave therapy in the rate at which men were catheter free at 6 months. Evidence was insufficient to draw conclusions for all other outcomes. Future research is necessary before information is useful in informing practice.
- We found no data to assess the impact of treating CUR independent of treating benign prostatic enlargement and other lower urinary tract symptoms.

We identified one systematic review and four studies that addressed treatments for CUR from non-obstructive causes. Evidence for all comparisons and primary outcomes was insufficient to draw conclusions about treatment, primarily because risk of bias was moderate and estimates were imprecise due to small sample sizes. The previous systematic review provides the highest level of evidence:

- Low-strength evidence suggested that sacral neuromodulation reduces the need for catheterization and PVR urine for CUR not attributable to obstructive causes.

Again, we found sparse data for analysis of treatments in populations with CUR from mixed obstructive/non-obstructive causes or from unknown causes. We identified only two eligible effectiveness studies and one relevant comparison in a previous systematic review. Evidence was insufficient for all comparisons and outcomes. Harms were inconsistently reported and studies were not powered to detect differences in those reported.

Applicability

The applicability or generalizability of our conclusions applies to patients with conditions similar to those examined in the eligible studies. Eligible studies did not address all possible populations in which CUR is common. Age and sex of subjects appear similar to the populations experiencing CUR from those causes in practice. Recruitment methods varied but were overall judged as likely to represent their respective populations. Conclusions lacked strength due to limited evidence, but participants in the eligible studies reflected the populations they represented.

Limitations

This review suffers from several limitations. First, we identified few studies that specifically evaluated treatments for CUR or that enrolled patient with CUR. Included studies often evaluated treatments for the underlying condition, such as benign prostatic enlargement and urinary symptoms. Treatments were similar to those used in the broader population (same conditions with only a subpopulation that suffers from CUR).

Many of the identified studies suffered from methodological weaknesses and were underpowered.

Future Research Needs

Our review provides low-strength evidence at best on a select few treatments for CUR attributed to a variety of underlying conditions. Evidence for most comparisons and outcomes was insufficient, demonstrating large gaps in the research on this topic. Although several ongoing studies (Appendix J) may, when completed, help close some of the gaps, additional research is also needed (specific recommendations appear in Appendix K).

Clarification or agreement on conceptual issues may help direct future research. Improved understanding of the natural history of CUR would provide context. It is not clear whether research on CUR should occur within underlying conditions or across conditions as this review attempted. Resolving these contextual issues would benefit future comparative effectiveness research.

A stronger comparative effectiveness evidence base will also require additional research. Many population groups known to suffer from CUR were not addressed by controlled studies. These include individuals with other obstructive or anatomical causes such as strictures or prolapsed organs, those with neurologic disorders such as diabetes mellitus, diabetic neuropathy, and Parkinson's disease, and women with CUR arising as a complication from surgery for stress urinary incontinence. Additionally, treatments other than those examined in included studies are available and may alleviate CUR. Pharmaceutical interventions are commonly used in men with BPH and evidence from those trials suggests that alpha-blockers help to reduce PVR volumes in men with BPH.[23] One study addressing this question is registered with ClinicalTrials.gov; however, results are not available.

Conclusions

Standard clinical diagnostic criteria are lacking for CUR, and the condition is variably defined in research. Because CUR is typically caused by other medical conditions, treatment options differ based on the underlying problem. The evidence addresses only a subset of possible treatments and just a few of the many possible subgroups of CUR patients based on underlying conditions. In men with bladder outlet obstruction from benign prostatic enlargement, TURP and microwave therapy achieved similar catheter-free rates at 6 months post treatment. However, because evidence on other outcomes was insufficient, we do not know the sustainability of benefits compared for these groups. Therefore, evidence on longer term outcomes is necessary to fully understand this comparison. Evidence on harms was not adequately powered to detect differences between groups. Therefore, these results are not useful in informing practice. We could not determine what portion of the improvement in primary outcomes is attributable to treating CUR (above and beyond treating the underlying condition). Treatment benefits likely result from improvements in lower urinary tract symptoms. In patients with CUR from non-obstructive causes, botulinum injections do not appear to reduce PVR urine volumes. In Fowler's syndrome patients, sacral neuromodulation may be effective. Data on treatment of "asymptomatic" patients with CUR was not informative because the population was not adequately defined.

References

1. Kaplan SA, Wein AJ, Staskin DR, et al. Urinary retention and post-void residual urine in men: separating truth from tradition. Journal of Urology. 2008 Jul;180(1):47-54. PMID: 18485378.
2. Negro CLA, Muir GH. Chronic urinary retention in men: How we define it, and how does it affect treatment outcome. BJU international. 2012.
3. Selius BA, Subedi R. Urinary retention in adults: diagnosis and initial management. American Family Physician. 2008 Mar 1;77(5):643-50. PMID: 18350762.
4. Yoshimura N, Chancellor MB. Differential diagnosis and treatment of impaired bladder emptying. Reviews in urology. 2004;6(Suppl 1):S24.
5. DasGupta R, Fowler CJ. The management of female voiding dysfunction: Fowler's syndrome -- a contemporary update. Current Opinion in Urology. 2003 Jul;13(4):293-9. PMID: 12811293.
6. Scottish Intercollegiate Guidelines Network. Search Filters. 2013. www.sign.ac.uk/methodology/filters.html. Accessed on July 23 2013.
7. White C, Ip S, McPheeters M, et al. Using existing systematic reviews to replace de novo processes in conducting Comparative Effectiveness Reviews. Agency for Healthcare Research and Quality. Rockville, MD: 2009. http://effectivehealthcare.ahrq.gov/repFiles/methodsguide/systematicreviewsreplacedenovo.pdf.
8. Agency for Healthcare Research and Quality. Grading the strength of a body of evidence when assessing health care interventions--AHRQ and the effective health-care program: An Update Draft Report. Rockville, MD: June 2012. http://effectivehealthcare.ahrq.gov/search-for-guides-reviews-and-reports/?pageaction=displayproduct&productid=1163
9. Atkins D, Chang S, Gartlehner G, et al. Assessing the Applicability of Studies When Comparing Medical Interventions. 2010. www.effectivehealthcare.ahrq.gov/index.cfm/search-for-guides-reviews-and-reports/?pageaction=displayProduct&productID=603#2412. Accessed on AHRQ Publication No. 11-EHC019-EF.
10. Datta SN, Kavia RB, Gonzales G, et al. Results of double-blind placebo-controlled crossover study of sildenafil citrate (Viagra) in women suffering from obstructed voiding or retention associated with the primary disorder of sphincter relaxation (Fowler's Syndrome). European Urology. 2007 Feb;51(2):489-95; discussion 95-7. PMID: 16884844.
11. Tang MW, Kwok TC, Hui E, et al. Intermittent versus indwelling urinary catheterization in older female patients. Maturitas. 2006 Feb 20;53(3):274-81. PMID: 16084677.
12. Schelin S, Geertsen U, Walter S, et al. Feedback microwave thermotherapy versus TURP/prostate enucleation surgery in patients with benign prostatic hyperplasia and persistent urinary retention: a prospective, randomized, controlled, multicenter study. Urology. 2006 Oct;68(4):795-9. PMID: 17070355.
13. Ghalayini IF, Al-Ghazo MA, Pickard RS. A prospective randomized trial comparing transurethral prostatic resection and clean intermittent self-catheterization in men with chronic urinary retention. BJU International. 2005 Jul;96(1):93-7. PMID: 15963128.
14. Gallien P, Reymann JM, Amarenco G, et al. Placebo controlled, randomised, double blind study of the effects of botulinum A toxin on detrusor sphincter dyssynergia in multiple sclerosis patients. Journal of Neurology, Neurosurgery & Psychiatry. 2005 Dec;76(12):1670-6. PMID: 16291892.
15. Hindley RG, Brierly RD, Thomas PJ. Prostaglandin E2 and bethanechol in combination for treating detrusor underactivity. BJU International. 2004 Jan;93(1):89-92. PMID: 14678375.
16. Chen YH, Kuo HC. Botulinum A toxin treatment of urethral sphincter pseudodyssynergia in patients with cerebrovascular accidents or intracranial lesions. Urologia Internationalis. 2004;73(2):156-61; discussion 61-2. PMID: 15331901.
17. de Seze M, Petit H, Gallien P, et al. Botulinum a toxin and detrusor sphincter dyssynergia: a double-blind lidocaine-controlled study in 13 patients with spinal cord disease. European Urology. 2002 Jul;42(1):56-62. PMID: 12121731.
18. Jonas U, Fowler CJ, Chancellor MB, et al. Efficacy of sacral nerve stimulation for urinary retention: results 18 months after implantation. Journal of Urology. 2001 Jan;165(1):15-9. PMID: 11125353.

19. Gujral S, Abrams P, Donovan JL, et al. A prospective randomized trial comparing transurethral resection of the prostate and laser therapy in men with chronic urinary retention: The CLasP study. Journal of Urology. 2000 Jul;164(1):59-64. PMID: 10840425.
20. Duffy LM, Cleary J, Ahern S, et al. Clean intermittent catheterization: safe, cost-effective bladder management for male residents of VA nursing homes. Journal of the American Geriatrics Society. 1995 Aug;43(8):865-70. PMID: 7636093.
21. Herbison GP, Arnold EP. Sacral neuromodulation with implanted devices for urinary storage and voiding dysfunction in adults. Cochrane Database of Systematic Reviews. 2009(2):CD004202. PMID: 19370596.
22. Moore Katherine N, Fader M, Getliffe K. Long-term bladder management by intermittent catheterisation in adults and children. John Wiley & Sons, Ltd; 2007. http://onlinelibrary.wiley.com/doi/10.1002/14651858.CD006008.pub2/abstract. Accessed on 4.
23. McNeill SA, Hargreave TB, Geffriaud-Ricouard C, et al. Postvoid residual urine in patients with lower urinary tract symptoms suggestive of benign prostatic hyperplasia: pooled analysis of eleven controlled studies with alfuzosin. Urology. 2001 Mar;57(3):459-65. PMID: 11248620.

Abbreviations

AUR	Acute urinary retention
BPH	Benign prostate hyperplasia
CI	Confidence interval
CISC	Clean intermittent self-catheterization
CUR	Chronic urinary retention
DSD	Detrusor sphincter dyssynergia
IPSS	International Prostate Symptom Score
LUTS	Lower urinary tract symptoms
MD	Mean difference
MS	Multiple sclerosis
NA	Not assessed
NR	Not reported
NS	No statistical difference
PICOTS	Population, interventions, comparison, outcomes, timing, setting
PVR	Post void residual
QoL	Quality of life
RCT	Randomized controlled trial
RR	Risk ratio
SR	Systematic review
TURP	Transurethral resection of the prostate
TWOC	Trial without catheter
UTI	Urinary tract infection

Appendix A. CUR Treatments

Table A1. Treatments for chronic urinary retention

Intervention	Type or Class
Catheterization	In-dwelling catheterization, intermittent catheterization (clean or sterile technique)
Surgical interventions (etiology-specific)	Male-specific etiologies: prostate surgeries Female-specific etiologies: pelvic organ prolapse repair, adjustment to stress urinary incontinence (SUI) procedures Nonsex-specific etiologies: sacral nerve stimulation, urethroplasty Multiple etiologies: urinary diversion procedures
Pharmacological interventions	Alpha blockers (AB) (doxazosin, prazosin, tamsulosin, terazosin, alfuzosin, silodosin); 5-Alpha Reductase Inhibitors (5-ARI): dutasteride, finasteride; AB + 5-ARI combination therapy: tamsulosin/dutasteride Neurogenic etiologies: botulinum toxin

AB = alpha blockers; SUI = stress urinary incontinence; 5-ARI = 5-alpha reductase inhibitors

Appendix B. Analytical Framework

Figure B1. Analytical framework

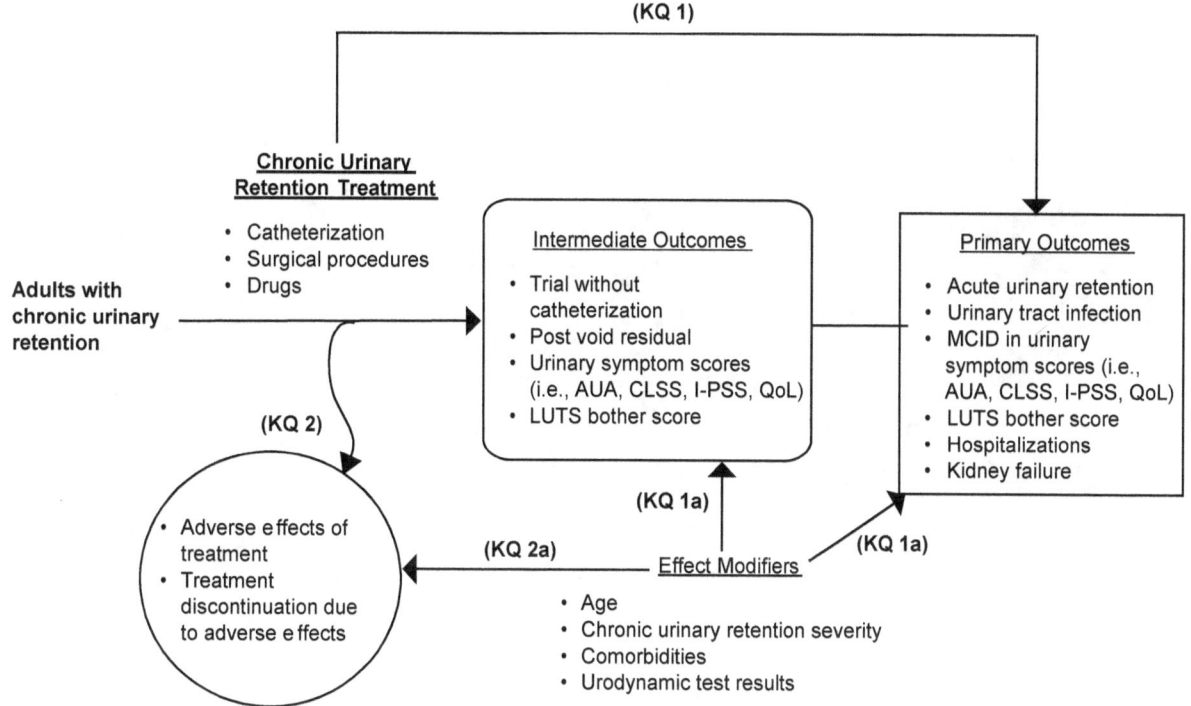

Appendix C. Search Strategy

MEDLINE

Database: Ovid MEDLINE(R) <1946 to November Week 3 2012> Search Strategy:

1. exp *Urinary Retention/ (1930)
2. "urinary retention".ti,ab. (5318)
3. "voiding dysfunction".ti,ab. (1312)
4. "incomplete voiding".ti,ab. (50)
5. "voiding difficult*".ti,ab. (423)
6. "underactive bladder".ti,ab. (27)
7. "incomplete bladder empt*".ti,ab. (117)
8. "elevated post void residual".ti,ab. (13)
9. ischuria.ti,ab. (29)
10. or/1-9 (7624)
11. limit 10 to "all child (0 to 18 years)" (1408)
12. limit 11 to "all adult (19 plus years)" (560)
13. 10 not 11 (6216)
14. 12 or 13 (6776)
15. limit 14 to animals (370)
16. 14 not 15 (6406)
17. Randomized Controlled Trials as Topic/ (84921)
18. randomized controlled trial/ (342334)
19. Random Allocation/ (76596)
20. Double Blind Method/ (118498)
21. Single Blind Method/ (17086)
22. clinical trial/ (476450)
23. clinical trial, phase i.pt. (12809)
24. clinical trial, phase ii.pt. (20505)
25. clinical trial, phase iii.pt. (7571)
26. clinical trial, phase iv.pt. (759)
27. controlled clinical trial.pt. (85694)
28. randomized controlled trial.pt. (342334)
29. multicenter study.pt. (153247)
30. clinical trial.pt. (476450)
31. exp Clinical Trials as topic/ (264416)
32. or/17-31 (949526)
33. (clinical adj trial$).tw. (178736)
34. ((singl$ or doubl$ or treb$ or tripl$) adj (blind$3 or mask$3)).tw. (116076)
35. PLACEBOS/ (31583)
36. placebo$.tw. (141131)
37. randomly allocated.tw. (14209)
38. (allocated adj2 random$).tw. (16559)
39. 33 or 34 or 35 or 36 or 37 or 38 (363492)
40. Epidemiologic studies/ (5579)
41. exp case control studies/ (586243)
42. exp cohort studies/ (1234174)
43. Case control.tw. (63924)
44. (cohort adj (study or studies)).tw. (65854)
45. Cohort analy$.tw. (2895)
46. (Follow up adj (study or studies)).tw. (33920)
47. (observational adj (study or studies)).tw. (33241)
48. Longitudinal.tw. (115334)
49. Retrospective.tw. (223737)
50. Cross sectional.tw. (130903)

51 Cross-sectional studies/ (150828)
52 40 or 41 or 42 or 43 or 44 or 45 or 46 or 47 or 48 or 49 or 50 or 51 (1654583)
53 Meta-Analysis as Topic/ (12608)
54 meta analy$.tw. (43811)
55 metaanaly$.tw. (1130)
56 Meta-Analysis/ (37918)
57 (systematic adj (review$1 or overview$1)).tw. (35503)
58 exp Review Literature as Topic/ (6626)
59 or/53-58 (89518)
60 32 or 39 or 52 or 59 (2503667)
61 16 and 60 (2820)

Note: a search with similar concept terms was used for the Cochrane Central Register of Controlled Trials.

Appendix D. Inclusion Criteria

Table D1. Study inclusion criteria

Category	Criteria for Inclusion
Study enrollment	Studies that enroll adults with CUR and test the effectiveness of treatments for CUR.
Study design	Meta-analyses, systematic reviews, RCTs, and nonrandomized controlled trials for each population and treatment option. Controlled before and after studies for KQs that cannot be answered using trial data alone.
Time of publication	Search all literature from 1946 forward.
Study quality	For all studies meeting inclusion criteria after title and abstract review, the full articles were screened for eligibility; studies of any risk of bias level were included.
Language of publication	Given that literature on this topic published in English best represents interventions available and accessible in the United States, we limited inclusion to studies with full text published in English. However, we did not limit our search based on language so that potential language bias could be assessed.

CUR = chronic urinary retention; KQ = key question; RCT = randomized controlled trial

Appendix E. Excluded Studies

Original Research Excluded

Yi WM, Pan AZ, Li JJ, et al. Clinical observation on the acupuncture treatment in patients with urinary retention after radical hysterectomy. Chinese Journal of Integrative Medicine. 2011 Nov;17(11):860-3. PMID 21809126. *Not CUR population*

Hakvoort RA, Thijs SD, Bouwmeester FW, et al. Comparing clean intermittent catheterisation and transurethral indwelling catheterisation for incomplete voiding after vaginal prolapse surgery: a multicentre randomised trial. BJOG: An International Journal of Obstetrics & Gynaecology. 2011 Aug;118(9):1055-60. PMID 21481147. *Not CUR population*

Chartier-Kastler E, Lauge I, Ruffion A, et al. Safety of a new compact catheter for men with neurogenic bladder dysfunction: a randomised, crossover and open-labelled study. Spinal Cord. 2011 Jul;49(7):844-50. PMID 21339763. *Not CUR population*

Autorino R, Damiano R, Di Lorenzo G, et al. Four-year outcome of a prospective randomised trial comparing bipolar plasmakinetic and monopolar transurethral resection of the prostate. European Urology. 2009 Apr;55(4):922-9. PMID 19185975. *Not CUR population*

Bjerklund Johansen T, Hultling C, Madersbacher H, et al. A novel product for intermittent catheterisation: its impact on compliance with daily life--international multicentre study. European Urology. 2007 Jul;52(1):213-20. PMID 17166653. *Not eligible study design*

Yamanishi T, Yasuda K, Kamai T, et al. Combination of a cholinergic drug and an alpha-blocker is more effective than monotherapy for the treatment of voiding difficulty in patients with underactive detrusor. International Journal of Urology. 2004 Feb;11(2):88-96. PMID 14706012. *Not CUR population*

McNeill SA, Hargreave TB, Geffriaud-Ricouard C, et al. Postvoid residual urine in patients with lower urinary tract symptoms suggestive of benign prostatic hyperplasia: pooled analysis of eleven controlled studies with alfuzosin. Urology. 2001 Mar;57(3):459-65. PMID 11248620. *Not CUR population*

Bernier F, Davila GW. The treatment of nonobstructive urinary retention with high-frequency transvaginal electrical stimulation. Urologic Nursing. 2000 Aug;20(4):261-4. PMID 11998089. *Not eligible study design*

Lukkarinen O, Hellstrom P, Leppilahti M, et al. Antibiotic prophylaxis in patients with urinary retention undergoing transurethral prostatectomy. Annales Chirurgiae et Gynaecologiae. 1997;86(3):239-42. PMID 9435936. *Not a treatment for CUR*

Belzner S. [Eucalyptus oil dressings in urinary retention]. Pflege Aktuell. 1997 Jun;51(6):386-7. PMID 9287850. *Not available in English*

Mompo Sanchis JA, Paya Navarro JJ, Prosper Rovira F. [Transurethral thermotherapy with microwaves in patients with benign prostatic hypertrophy and urinary retention: comparative study between high energy (25) and standard energy (2.0)]. Archivos Espanoles de Urologia. 1996 May;49(4):337-46. PMID 8754190. *Not available in English*

King RB, Carlson CE, Mervine J, et al. Clean and sterile intermittent catheterization methods in hospitalized patients with spinal cord injury. Archives of Physical Medicine & Rehabilitation. 1992 Sep;73(9):798-802. PMID 1514886. *Not CUR population*

Abrams PH, Shah PJ, Gaches CG, et al. Role of suprapubic catheterization in retention of urine. Journal of the Royal Society of Medicine. 1980 Dec;73(12):845-8. PMID 7005439. *Not CUR population*

Systematic Reviews Excluded

Barendrecht MM, Oelke M, Laguna MP, et al. Is the use of parasympathomimetics for treating an underactive urinary bladder evidence-based? BJU International. 2007 Apr;99(4):749-52. PMID 17233798. *Not Relevant*

Chartier-Kastler E, Denys P. Intermittent catheterization with hydrophilic catheters as a treatment of chronic neurogenic urinary retention. Neurourology & Urodynamics. 2011 Jan;30(1):21-31. PMID 20928913. *Not SR*

Getliffe K, Fader M, Allen C, et al. Current evidence on intermittent catheterization: sterile single-use catheters or clean reused catheters and the incidence of UTI. Journal of Wound, Ostomy, & Continence Nursing. 2007 May-Jun;34(3):289-96. PMID 17505249. *Not Relevant*

Hagen S, Stark D. Conservative prevention and management of pelvic organ prolapse in women. John Wiley & Sons, Ltd. 2011. http://onlinelibrary.wiley.com/doi/10.1002/14651858.CD003882.pub4/abstract. *Not Relevant*

Jahn P, Beutner K, Langer G. Types of indwelling urinary catheters for long-term bladder drainage in adults. John Wiley & Sons, Ltd; 2012. http://onlinelibrary.wiley.com/doi/10.1002/14651858.CD004997.pub3/abstract. *Not Relevant*

Jamison J, Maguire S, McCann J. Catheter policies for management of long term voiding problems in adults with neurogenic bladder disorders. John Wiley & Sons, Ltd; 2011. http://onlinelibrary.wiley.com/doi/10.1002/14651858.CD004375.pub3/abstract. *Not Relevant*

Lefevre F, Civic D, Aronson N, et al. Percutaneous tibial nerve stimulation for the treatment of voiding dysfunction. Technology Evaluation Center Assessment Program. 2011 Mar;25(8):1-7. PMID 21638944. *Not Relevant*

Mehta S, Hill D, Foley N, et al. A meta-analysis of botulinum toxin sphincteric injections in the treatment of incomplete voiding after spinal cord injury. Archives of Physical Medicine & Rehabilitation. 2012 Apr;93(4):597-603. PMID 22365478. *Not Relevant*

Moore KN, Burt J, Voaklander DC. Itermittent catheterization in the rehabilitation setting: a comparison of clean and sterile technique. Clinical rehabilitation. 2006;20(6):461-8. *Not Relevant*

Utomo E, Blok B. Surgical management of functional bladder outlet obstruction in adults with neurogenic bladder dysfunction. John Wiley & Sons, Ltd; 2011. http://onlinelibrary.wiley.com/doi/10.1002/14651858.CD004927.pub3/abstract. *Not Relevant*

Appendix F. Description and Characteristics of Included Studies

Table F1. Characteristics of included studies

Author, Year, Funding, Design	Inclusion/Exclusion Criteria	Patient Characteristics	CUR Characteristics	CUR Urodynamics/ Severity (Expressed in means unless noted)	Risk of Bias
Datta, 2007[1] UK Grant RCT N=20	Inclusion criteria: women aged 18-65 year suffering with complete or partial retention or obstructive voiding. Exclusion criteria: major hematologic, renal, or hepatic impairment and major psychiatric disorders not well controlled by treatment; significant cardiovascular disease and a history of stroke or myocardial infarction in the previous 6 months; resting blood pressure over 90/50mmHg and 180/110 mmHg; known history of retinitis pigmentosa; uses of nitrates or NO donors	Age, mean: 39 Gender: women 100% Race: NR Comorbidities: NR Intervention: sildenafil citrate Control: placebo	Definition/etiology max flow rate <15ml/min, max urethral closure pressure 92-age cmH_2O, sphincter volume >1.6 cm^3 Fowler's syndrome Concurrent treatment: NR Previous treatments: NR	PVR (ml): 140 IPSS: 21.5 MUCP (cmH_2O): 106.6 Sphincter volume (cm^3): 2.1 Detrusor pressure at qmax (cmH_2O): 35.2 Voiding time (sec): 90.5	Overall risk of bias: medium
Schelin, 2006[2] Sweden, Denmark, and Norway Not reported RCT N=120	Inclusion criteria: patients ≥45 years, with symptomatic BPH and persistent urinary retention requiring an indwelling catheter or clean intermittent catheterization for at least 1 month before screening. Exclusion criteria: Patients who were medically and/or psychologically unable to tolerate surgery	Intervention: ProstaLund feedback treatment n=61 Age, mean: 73 Gender: men 100% Race: NR Comorbidities: NR Control: TURP or prostate enucleation surgery n=59 Age, mean: 73 Gender: men 100% Race: NR Comorbidities: NR	Definition/etiology: PVR ≥300 ml BPH Concurrent treatment: NR Previous treatments: NR	Intervention: PLFT Indwelling catheter: 87% Catheterization Control: TURP and prostate enucleation surgery Indwelling catheter: 86% Catheterization	Overall risk of bias: medium
Tang, 2006[3] Hong Kong, China Not reported RCT N=81	Inclusion criteria: female patients ≥65 years of age admitted to a female geriatric rehabilitation ward with PVR over ≥300 ml on two occasions Exclusion criteria: terminally ill or those who required an indwelling urinary catheter for	Intervention: intermittent urinary catheterization n=36 Age, mean: 80 Gender: women 100% Race: NR	Definition/etiology PVR persistently ≥300 ml Concurrent treatment: diuretics: 25%	Intervention: PVR (ml): 545.9 Past history of urinary retention: 6% Control: PVR (ml): 539.8	Overall risk of bias: medium

Author, Year, Funding, Design	Inclusion/Exclusion Criteria	Patient Characteristics	CUR Characteristics	CUR Urodynamics/ Severity (Expressed in means unless noted)	Risk of Bias
	urine output monitoring.	Mean Barthel index (baseline disability) (out of 20): 7.8 Comorbidities: NR Control: indwelling urinary catheterization n=45 Age, mean: 81 Gender: women 100% Race: NR Mean Barthel index (baseline disability) (out of 20): 6.2 Comorbidities: NR	calcium channel blockers: 11% anticholinergic agents:19% alpha-blockers: 3% distigmine bromide: 0% Previous treatments: NR	Past history of urinary retention: 0%	
Gallien, 2005[4] France Not for profit organizations RCT N=86	Inclusion criteria: Patients >18 years of age and suffering from MS with DSD. The diagnosis of MS had to have been made according to Poser criteria at least 6 months before inclusion Exclusion criteria: Urine or prostate febrile infection, perineal skin disorders, or myasthenia, or if they took any treatment which could have altered neuromuscular transmission. Pregnant women or non-menopausal women who did not take effective contraception were also excluded.	Intervention: botulinum A toxin n=45 Age, mean: 50 Gender: men 38% Race: NR Expanded disability status scale: 5.4 Comorbidities: NR Time from onset of urinary disorders (months): 98 Incontinence: 78% Control: placebo n=41 Age, mean: 51 Gender: men 27% Race: NR Expanded disability status scale: 6.0 Comorbidities: NR Time from onset of urinary disorders (months): 111 Incontinence: 83%	Definition/etiology: Patients with CUR were included if they had PVR between 100 and 500 ml. Concurrent treatment: Patients were prescribed an alpha blocker (5 mg tablet of slow release alfuzosin bid) over 4 months. Previous treatments: Alpha blocker use before inclusion: 56%	Intervention: botulinum A toxin PVR (ml): 220 Peak urine flow(ml/s): 13 IPSS: 21 Voiding volume (ml): 135 Blaivas's classification of DSD: Type 2: 40% Type 3: 44% Control: placebo PVR (ml): 217 Peak urine flow (ml/s): 16 IPSS: 20 Voiding volume (ml): 166 Blaivas's classification of DSD: Type 2: 34% Type 3: 44%	Overall risk of bias: medium

Author, Year, Funding, Design	Inclusion/Exclusion Criteria	Patient Characteristics	CUR Characteristics	CUR Urodynamics/ Severity (Expressed in means unless noted)	Risk of Bias
Ghalayini, 2005[5] Jordan Not reported RCT N=41	Inclusion criteria: men with LUTS and an IPSS of >7, together with CUR, defined as a PVR of >300 ml measured by ultra-sonography on two occasions, with patients and physicians agreeing that the findings justified intervention. Exclusion criteria: clinical evidence of prostate cancer, infection, previous prostatic surgery, uncontrolled renal impairment, a life-expectancy of <6 months, proven neurological bladder dysfunction, or inability to practice CISC.	Intervention: transurethral resection of the prostate (TURP) n=17 Age, mean: 67 Gender: men 100% Race: NR Comorbidities: NR Control: Clean intermittent self-catheterization (CISC) n=24 Age, mean: 69 Gender: men 100% Race: NR Comorbidities: NR	Definition/etiology: PVR of >300 ml Concurrent treatment: All had a 4-6-week period of indwelling catheterization to stabilize renal function before starting the allocated management Previous treatments: NR	Intervention: IPSS: 25.8 IPSS QoL: 4.4 PVR (ml): 954 Control: IPSS: 23.2 IPSS QoL: 4.2 PVR (ml): 963	Overall risk of bias: medium
Chen, 2004[6] Taiwan, China Grant Prospective study	Inclusion criteria: Patients with chronic cerebrovascular accidents or intracranial lesions were enrolled. All patients had symptoms of severe difficulty in initiation of urination or urinary retention. Exclusion criteria: NR	N=21 Intervention: botulinum A toxin n=11 Age, mean: 67 Gender: men 45% Race: NR Comorbidities: Stroke: 73% Intracranial hemorrhage:18% Meningitis: 9% Detrusor hyperreflexia: 91% Detrusor underactivity: 9% Urethral sphincter pseudodyssynergia: 100% Control: usual care n=10 Age, mean: 65	Definition/etiology: NR Concurrent treatment: NR Previous treatments: Medications such as α-blockers, skeletal muscle relaxants, or nitric oxide donors without remarkable effect.	Intervention: PVR (ml): 126 IPSS: 27.3 QoL: 4.7 Control: PVR (ml): NR IPSS: 22.5 QoL: 4.3	Overall risk of bias: medium

Author, Year, Funding, Design	Inclusion/Exclusion Criteria	Patient Characteristics	CUR Characteristics	CUR Urodynamics/ Severity (Expressed in means unless noted)	Risk of Bias
		Gender: men 70% Race: NR Comorbidities: Stroke: 100% Detrusor hyperreflexia: 80% Detrusor underactivity: 20%			
Hindley 2004[7] UK Not reported RCT N=19	Inclusion criteria: Patients with suspected detrusor underactivity. Exclusion criteria: Asthma, hyperthyroidism, severe bradycardia, hypotension, recent myocardial infarction, bowel obstruction, active peptic ulcer disease, epilepsy, parkinsonism and evidence of serious concomitant psychiatric disease. Patients who were categorized as obstructed on the nomogram were also excluded from the study (all patients had an Abrams-Griffiths number of <40).	Intervention: bethanechol chloride (BC) plus prostaglandin E2 (PGE2) n=9 Age, mean: 67 Gender: men 89% Race: NR Comorbidities: bladder neck incision: 22% TURP: 33% interstitial radiofrequency therapy to the prostate: 11% chronic retention: 11% Control: placebo n=10 Age, mean: 64 Gender: men 90% Race: NR Comorbidities: Bladder neck incision: 10% TURP: 30% Chronic retention: 40%	Definition/etiology: PVR consistently >300ml in the absence of BOO. Concurrent treatment: NR Previous treatments: NR	Intervention: Frequency of CISC/day: 2.22 CISC volume drained (ml): 381.25 PVR (ml), median: 426 Control: Frequency of CISC/day: 2.70 CISC volume drained (ml): 505 PVR (ml), median: 575.5	Overall risk of bias: medium
de Sèze, 2002[8] France The Coloplast Foundation for quality of life RCT	Inclusion criteria: presence of DSD in patients affected by upper motor neuron type bladder dysfunction due to medical (MS, myelitis) or traumatic spinal disease which was neurologically stable (i.e., no progression in neurological symptoms in the previous 3	Intervention: botulinum A toxin n=5 Age, mean: 41 Gender: men 80% Race: NR	Definition/etiology: PVR >100 ml Concurrent treatment: No concurrent treatments	Intervention: PVR (ml): 264.4 MUP (cmH$_2$O): 109.4 Blaivas's classification of DSD: Type 3: 40%	Overall risk of bias: medium

Author, Year, Funding, Design	Inclusion/Exclusion Criteria	Patient Characteristics	CUR Characteristics	CUR Urodynamics/ Severity (Expressed in means unless noted)	Risk of Bias
N=13	months). Exclusion criteria: pregnancy, blood coagulation, abnormalities, inflammation or infection of the injection site, myasthenia, aminoglycoside treatment, hypersensitivity to botulinum toxin or lidocaine, lidocaine contraindications and lower motor neuron perineal lesion.	Comorbidities: Spinal cord injury: 80% MS: 20% Control: lidocaine n=8 Age, mean: 49 Gender: men 100% Race: NR Comorbidities: Spinal cord injury: 63% MS: 25% Dural fistulization: 12.5%	Previous treatments: NR	Type 2: 40% Type 1: 20% DP (cmH_2O): 74.2 Control: PRV (ml): 313.1 MUP (cmH_2O): 83.2 Blaivas's classification of DSD: Type 3: 38% Type 2: 62% DP (cmH_2O): 88.6	
Gujral, 2000[9] UK Government (NHS) RCT N=82	Inclusion criteria: LUTS with an IPSS) ≥8 indicating moderate to severe symptoms. Patients had a urinary flow rate of <15, <13, <10 ml/s when voided volume was >200, between 150 and 200, and between 100 and 149 ml, as measured on at least 2 occasions. Exclusion criteria: Clinically diagnosed prostate cancer, previous prostatic surgery, life expectancy <6 months, neuropathic bladder dysfunction, serum creatinine >250 mmol, abnormal upper tracts on renal tract ultrasonography or a prostate volume >120 cc, men on long-term active medication for the lower urinary tract.	Intervention: Transurethral prostatic resection n=44 Age, mean:71 Gender: men 100% Race: white 100% Comorbidities: NR Control: Laser therapy n=38 Age, mean: 70 Gender: men 100% Race: white 100% Comorbidities: NR	Definition/etiology: PVR >300 ml BPH Concurrent treatment: NR Previous treatments: NR	Intervention: PVR (ml): 545 IPSS: 19.5 IPSS quality of life score, median: 4.5 Peak urine flow (ml/s): 8.5 Control: Laser therapy PVR (ml): 438 IPSS: 20.9 IPSS quality of life score, median: 5.0 Peak urine flow (ml/s): 11.2	Overall risk of bias: medium

BOO = bladder outflow obstruction; BPH = benign prostatic hyperplasia; BPO = benign prostatic obstruction; CISC = clean intermittent self-catheterization; CUR = chronic urinary retention; DP = detrusor pressure; DSD = detrusor sphincter dyssynergia; IPSS = International Prostate Symptom Score; LUTS = lower urinary tract symptoms; MS = multiple sclerosis; MUCP = maximal urethral closure pressure; MUP = maximal urethral pressure; NR = not reported; PLFT = ProstaLund Feedback Treatment; PVR = post-voiding residual urine volume; TURP = transurethral resection of the prostate; UTI = urinary tract infection

References for Appendix F

1. Datta SN, Kavia RB, Gonzales G, et al. Results of double-blind placebo-controlled crossover study of sildenafil citrate (Viagra) in women suffering from obstructed voiding or retention associated with the primary disorder of sphincter relaxation (Fowler's Syndrome). European Urology. 2007 Feb;51(2):489-95; discussion 95-7. PMID 16884844.
2. Schelin S, Geertsen U, Walter S, et al. Feedback microwave thermotherapy versus TURP/prostate enucleation surgery in patients with benign prostatic hyperplasia and persistent urinary retention: a prospective, randomized, controlled, multicenter study. Urology. 2006 Oct;68(4):795-9. PMID 17070355.
3. Tang MW, Kwok TC, Hui E, et al. Intermittent versus indwelling urinary catheterization in older female patients. Maturitas. 2006 Feb 20;53(3):274-81. PMID 16084677.
4. Gallien P, Reymann JM, Amarenco G, et al. Placebo controlled, randomised, double blind study of the effects of botulinum A toxin on detrusor sphincter dyssynergia in multiple sclerosis patients. Journal of Neurology, Neurosurgery & Psychiatry. 2005 Dec;76(12):1670-6. PMID 16291892.
5. Ghalayini IF, Al-Ghazo MA, Pickard RS. A prospective randomized trial comparing transurethral prostatic resection and clean intermittent self-catheterization in men with chronic urinary retention. BJU International. 2005 Jul;96(1):93-7. PMID 15963128.
6. Chen YH, Kuo HC. Botulinum A toxin treatment of urethral sphincter pseudodyssynergia in patients with cerebrovascular accidents or intracranial lesions. Urologia Internationalis. 2004;73(2):156-61; discussion 61-2. PMID 15331901.
7. Hindley RG, Brierly RD, Thomas PJ. Prostaglandin E2 and bethanechol in combination for treating detrusor underactivity. BJU International. 2004 Jan;93(1):89-92. PMID 14678375.
8. de Seze M, Petit H, Gallien P, et al. Botulinum a toxin and detrusor sphincter dyssynergia: a double-blind lidocaine-controlled study in 13 patients with spinal cord disease. European Urology. 2002 Jul;42(1):56-62. PMID 12121731.
9. Gujral S, Abrams P, Donovan JL, et al. A prospective randomized trial comparing transurethral resection of the prostate and laser therapy in men with chronic urinary retention: The CLasP study. Journal of Urology. 2000 Jul;164(1):59-64. PMID 10840425.

Appendix G. Risk of Bias and Quality

Table G1. Risk of bias of included original research

Study	Outcome	Risk of Selection Bias Due to Inadequate Randomization	Risk of Selection Bias Due to Inadequate Allocation	Risk of Performance Bias Due to Inadequate Blinding of Provider and Patient	Risk of Detection Bias Due to Inadequate Blinding	Risk of Attrition Bias	Risk of Reporting Bias Due to Selective Outcome Reporting	Intent To Treat	Groups Similar at Baseline	Other Risks of Bias	Overall Risk of Bias per Study-Outcome
RCTs											
Datta 2007[1]	UTI	Unclear	Unclear	Low	Unclear	Low	Low	Yes	Yes	No	Moderate
	IPSS	Unclear	Unclear	Low	Unclear	Low	Low	Yes	Yes	No	Moderate
	PVR	Unclear	Unclear	Low	Unclear	Low	Low	Yes	Yes	No	Moderate
Schelin 2006[2]	UTI	Unclear	High	High	Unclear	Low	Low	Unclear	Yes	No	Moderate
	Cath Free	Unclear	High	High	Unclear	Low	Low	Unclear	Yes	No	Moderate
	IPSS	Unclear	High	High	Unclear	Low	Low	Unclear	Yes	No	Moderate
	IPSS QoL	Unclear	High	High	Unclear	Low	Low	Unclear	Yes	No	Moderate
Tang 2006[3]	UTI	Low	Unclear	High	High	Low	Low	Yes	Yes	No	Moderate
	TWOC	Low	Unclear	High	High	Low	Low	Yes	Yes	No	Moderate
	PVR	Low	Unclear	High	High	Low	Low	Yes	Yes	No	Moderate
Gallien 2005[4]	UTI	Low	Low	Low	Unclear	Low	Low	Yes	Yes	Yes	Moderate
	IPSS	Low	Low	Low	Unclear	Low	Low	Yes	Yes	Yes	Moderate
	PVR	Low	Low	Low	Unclear	Low	Low	Yes	Yes	Yes	Moderate
Ghalayini 2005[5]	IPSS	High	Unclear	High	High	Low	Low	Yes	No	No	Moderate
	PVR	High	Unclear	High	High	Low	Low	Yes	No	No	Moderate
Hindley 2004[6]	QoL	High	Unclear	Low	Unclear	Low	Low	Yes	No	No	High
	PVR	High	Unclear	Low	Unclear	Low	Low	Yes	No	No	Moderate
de Sèze 2002[7]	PVR	Low	Unclear	Low	Unclear	Low	Low	Yes	Yes	No	Moderate
Gujral 2000[8]	UTI	High	Low	High	Unclear	Low	Low	Yes	No	Yes	High
	IPSS Category, adjusted	High	Low	High	Unclear	Low	Low	Yes	No	No	Moderate
	PVR, adjusted	High	Low	High	Unclear	Low	Low	Yes	No	No	Moderate
Cohort											
Chen 2004[9]	IPSS	High	NA	NA	NA	NA	Low	Low	Unclear	Yes[1]	High
	IPSS QoL	High	NA	NA	NA	NA	Low	Low	Unclear	Yes[1]	High
	PVR	High	NA	NA	NA	NA	Low	Low	Unclear	Yes[1]	High

IPSS = International Prostate Symptom Score; PVR: post-void residual urine volume; QoL = quality of life.
[1] No adjustments for selection bias during analysis.

References for Table G1

1. Datta SN, Kavia RB, Gonzales G, et al. Results of double-blind placebo-controlled crossover study of sildenafil citrate (Viagra) in women suffering from obstructed voiding or retention associated with the primary disorder of sphincter relaxation (Fowler's Syndrome). European Urology. 2007 Feb;51(2):489-95; discussion 95-7. PMID 16884844.
2. Schelin S, Geertsen U, Walter S, et al. Feedback microwave thermotherapy versus TURP/prostate enucleation surgery in patients with benign prostatic hyperplasia and persistent urinary retention: a prospective, randomized, controlled, multicenter study. Urology. 2006 Oct;68(4):795-9. PMID 17070355.
3. Tang MW, Kwok TC, Hui E, et al. Intermittent versus indwelling urinary catheterization in older female patients. Maturitas. 2006 Feb 20;53(3):274-81. PMID 16084677.
4. Gallien P, Reymann JM, Amarenco G, et al. Placebo controlled, randomised, double blind study of the effects of botulinum A toxin on detrusor sphincter dyssynergia in multiple sclerosis patients. Journal of Neurology, Neurosurgery & Psychiatry. 2005 Dec;76(12):1670-6. PMID 16291892.
5. Ghalayini IF, Al-Ghazo MA, Pickard RS. A prospective randomized trial comparing transurethral prostatic resection and clean intermittent self-catheterization in men with chronic urinary retention. BJU International. 2005 Jul;96(1):93-7. PMID 15963128.
6. Hindley RG, Brierly RD, Thomas PJ. Prostaglandin E2 and bethanechol in combination for treating detrusor underactivity. BJU International. 2004 Jan;93(1):89-92. PMID 14678375.
7. de Seze M, Petit H, Gallien P, et al. Botulinum a toxin and detrusor sphincter dyssynergia: a double-blind lidocaine-controlled study in 13 patients with spinal cord disease. European Urology. 2002 Jul;42(1):56-62. PMID 12121731.
8. Gujral S, Abrams P, Donovan JL, et al. A prospective randomized trial comparing transurethral resection of the prostate and laser therapy in men with chronic urinary retention: The CLasP study. Journal of Urology. 2000 Jul;164(1):59-64. PMID 10840425.
9. Chen YH, Kuo HC. Botulinum A toxin treatment of urethral sphincter pseudodyssynergia in patients with cerebrovascular accidents or intracranial lesions. Urologia Internationalis. 2004;73(2):156-61; discussion 61-2. PMID 15331901.

Table G2. Quality of previous systematic reviews

Study	A priori Study Design	Dual Study Selection and Data Abstraction	Comprehensive literature search	Publication Status	Lists of Included and Excluded Studies Provided?	Scientific Quality of Included Studies Assessed and Documented?	Scientific Quality of Included Studies Used Appropriately in Formulating Conclusions?	Methods of Combining Studies Appropriate?	Likelihood of Publication Bias Assessed?	Conflict of Interest Stated?	Overall Quality
Moore 2007[1]	yes	yes	yes	yes	yes	yes	yes	yes	Unclear	yes	good
Herbison 2009[2]	yes	yes	yes	yes	yes	yes	yes	yes	Unclear	yes	good

References for Table G2

1. Moore Katherine N, Fader M, Getliffe K. Long-term bladder management by intermittent catheterisation in adults and children. John Wiley & Sons, Ltd; 2007. http://onlinelibrary.wiley.com/doi/10.1002/14651858.CD006008.pub2/abstract. Accessed on 4.

2. Herbison GP, Arnold EP. Sacral neuromodulation with implanted devices for urinary storage and voiding dysfunction in adults. Cochrane Database of Systematic Reviews. 2009(2):CD004202. PMID 19370596.

Appendix H. Detailed Results

Contents

Comparative Effectiveness of Treatments for CUR: Obstructive Causes H-2
    Primary Outcomes H-2
    Intermediate Outcomes H-2
    Harms H-3
Comparative Effectiveness of Treatments for CUR: Non-Obstructive Causes H-8
    Primary Outcomes H-8
    Intermediate Outcomes H-8
    Harms H-8
Comparative Effectiveness of Treatments for CUR: Mixed Populations/Unknown Causes ... H-14
    Primary Outcomes H-14
    Intermediate Outcomes H-15
    Harms H-15
References for Appendix H H-18

Tables

Table H1 Comparative Effectiveness of Treatments for CUR from Obstructive Causes: summary of included studies H-4
Table H2 Comparative Effectiveness of Treatments for CUR from Obstructive Causes: primary outcomes H-5
Table H3 Comparative Effectiveness of Treatments for CUR from Obstructive Causes: intermediate outcomes H-6
Table H4 Comparative Effectiveness of Treatments for CUR from Obstructive Causes: adverse events H-7
Table H5 Description and Conclusions from Previous Systematic Reviews on Treatments for CUR from Non-obstructive Causes H-10
Table H6 Comparative Effectiveness of Treatments for CUR from Non-obstructive Causes: summary of included studies H-10
Table H7 Comparative Effectiveness of Treatments for CUR from Non-obstructive Causes: primary outcomes H-11
Table H8 Comparative Effectiveness of Treatments for CUR from Non-obstructive Causes: intermediate outcomes H-12
Table H9 Comparative Effectiveness of Treatments for CUR from Non-obstructive Causes: adverse events H-13
Table H10 Description and Conclusions from Previous Systematic Reviews on Treatments for CUR in Mixed Populations/Unknown Causes: H-16
Table H11 Comparative Effectiveness of Treatments for CUR in Mixed Populations/Unknown Causes: primary outcomes H-16
Table H12 Comparative Effectiveness of Treatments for CUR in Mixed Populations/Unknown Causes: intermediate outcomes H-17
Table H13 Comparative Effectiveness of Treatments for CUR in Mixed Populations/Unknown Causes: adverse events H-17

Comparative Effectiveness of Treatments for CUR: Obstructive Causes

We identified only three eligible studies comparing treatments for CUR from obstructive causes. Three eligible RCTs compared treatments for CUR in men with bladder outlet obstruction secondary to benign prostatic enlargement.[1-3] Each of these studies included men with CUR (defined as persistent PVR >300ml) and other lower urinary tract symptoms. Study and patient characteristics appear in Table H1. The mean age of the 243 men enrolled in these studies was 71. Two studies reported mean baseline IPSS scores and PVR volumes with a mean baseline total IPSS score of 21.4 (severe symptoms) and mean baseline PVR volume of 626 ml. All three trials compared surgery (transurethral resection of the prostate or prostate enucleation) to a less invasive intervention (laser, microwave, clean intermittent sterile catheterization). Two of these trials were conducted in Europe and one in Asia. All three RCTs demonstrated methodological problems (limited ability for blinding and allocation concealment) and each was assessed to have an overall medium risk of bias.

Primary Outcomes

Two of the three RCTs reported on five primary outcomes (UTI, treatment failure, trial without catheter [TWOC], need for surgical intervention, and IPSS category) (Table H2). The third RCT assessed only intermediate outcomes. We included IPSS category as a primary outcome because no study reported those achieving a minimum clinically important difference as the primary variable and the categorization better measures a clinical difference than changes in mean scores. Overall, the studies reported few differences in primary outcomes between groups, with both treatment groups typically showing improvements over baseline.

No studies reported AUR. Schelin et al. and Gujral et al. reported rates of UTI. More than 30 percent of the microwave therapy patients and 22 percent of the TURP patients experienced a UTI over the 6-month followup period.[3] UTI was recorded only as a postsurgical complication in the other study with nearly 5 percent of the TURP patients and nearly 3 percent of the laser therapy patients experiencing a postsurgical UTI.[2] Neither difference between treatment groups was statistically significant.

Gujral, et al. reported on surgical interventions. Three patients in the laser therapy group required TURP for continuing symptoms. None of the TURP patients needed to return to surgery; the difference was not statistically significant.[2] IPSS category was also measured in this study. Nearly 88 percent of the TURP patients and 69 percent of the laser therapy patients were in the good category after treatment. Once adjusted (groups differed at baseline in marital status and prostate volume), the proportional odds model indicated this difference was statistically significant favoring TURP (OR=3.9; CI: 1.0 to 14.3).

Intermediate Outcomes

Outcomes that we classified as intermediate were more frequently reported and authors may have considered them primary outcomes in their research (Table H3). Mean changes in continuous IPSS scores were reported in two of the three trials. When TURP is compared to clean intermittent self-catheterization, the TURP patients mean IPSS score improved by 20 points whereas the catheter patients mean score improved by 12 points. This level of change would be considered clinically important; however, confidence intervals were too wide for the difference to be statistically significant and included values that would not represent clinically meaningful change. Schelin, et al., report that after 3 months, the mean IPSS score in the microwave therapy group was 7.3 and 5.1 in the TURP/enucleation group[3]. At 6 months, these scores were 7.3 and 4.1, respectively.[3] This difference did not reach statistical significance nor are the values clinically important. The adjusted mean change in IPSS scores for the TURP versus laser therapy group was statistically significant after adjustment (adjusted mean difference = -3.6; CI: -7.2 to -0.1).[2] No other changes in intermediate outcomes (IPSS Quality of Life scores, PVR) were statistically significant for either comparison.

Harms

Each study measured adverse effects differently, reporting either the incidence of serious adverse effects or complication rates (Table H4). These harms did not differ between groups in the surgery versus microwave therapy or in surgery versus clean intermittent self-catheterization. However, a larger proportion of the TURP group experienced complications than the laser group. Strength of evidence was not assessed for harms.

Table H1. Comparative effectiveness of treatments for CUR from obstructive causes: summary of included studies

Number of studies	3
Randomized controlled trials	3
Number of patients enrolled (range)	243 (41 to 120)
Age of subjects, mean years (range)	71 (68 to 73)
Gender (range)	Men 100%
Baseline mean IPSS total score (range) (range 0 to 35)*	21.4 (20.0 to 24.3; 2 studies†)
Baseline mean PVR, mL (range)	626 (459 to 959; 2 studies†)
Neurogenic disease etiology	NR
Neurogenic disease duration, mean years	NR
Trials conducted in the United States (% of patients)	None
Trials conducted in Europe (% of patients)	2 (83)
Trials conducted in Asia (% of patients)	1 (17)
Studies reporting primary outcomes	2
Studies reporting secondary outcomes	3

* IPSS = International Prostate Symptom Score: Scoring criteria are: Mild (score 1-7); Moderate (score 8-19); Severe (score 20-35); NR = not reported; PVR=post-void residual

† Number of studies reporting this variable

Table H2. Comparative effectiveness of treatments for CUR from obstructive causes: primary outcomes

Study Design Followup	Treatment Arms	Acute Urinary Retention n/N (%)	Urinary Tract Infection n/N (%)	Surgical Intervention n/N (%)	IPSS* n/N (%)	Catheter Free n/N (%)
Schelin, 2006[3] RCT 6 months	TUMT (n=61)	NR	20/61 (32.8)	NR	NR	48/61†† (78.7)
	TURP or enucleation (n=59)	NR	13/59 (22)	NR	NR	52/59†† (88.1)
	RR [95% CI]		1.49 [0.82 to 2.71]			0.89 [0.76 to 1.05]
Ghalanyini, 2005[1] RCT 6 months	TURP (n=22)	NR	NR	NR	NR	NR
	CISC (n=29)	NR	NR	NR	NR	NR
	RR [95% CI]					
Gujral, 2000 RCT[2] 7.5 months	TURP (n=44)	NR	2/44 (4.5)	0/44	"good"† 29/33 (87.9)	NR
	Laser (n=38)	NR	1/38 (2.6)	3/38 (7.9)**	"good"† 20/29 (69.0)	NR
	RR [95% CI]		1.73 [0.16 to 18.31]	0.12 [0.01 to 2.32]	1.27 [0.97 to 1.68]	
	Adjusted OR		NR	NR	3.9 [1.0 to 14.3]	

CI = confidence interval; CISC = clean intermittent self-catheterization; IPSS = International Prostate Symptom Score (range 0 (mild symptoms) to 35 (severe symptoms); NR – not reported; RCT = randomized controlled trial; RR=risk ratio; TUMT = transurethral microwave therapy; TURP = transurethral resection of the prostate
* Subjects with clinically relevant improvement from baseline
** These patients required a TURP following laser surgery due to "unacceptable levels of symptoms."
† "Good" defined as postoperative score <8 or ≥50% reduction from baseline
†† All patients required catheterization at baseline

Table H3. Comparative effectiveness of treatments for CUR from obstructive causes: intermediate outcomes

Study; Design; Followup	Treatment Arms	IPSS, Mean (SD) at Baseline	IPSS, Mean (SD) Change from Baseline	IPSS QoL, Mean (SD) at Baseline	IPSS QoL, Mean Change (SD) from Baseline	PVR (mL), Mean (SD) at Baseline	PVR (mL), Mean (SD) Change from Baseline
Schelin, 2006[3] RCT 6 months	TUMT (n=61)	NR	7.3** (7.3) (n=50)	~4.6† [3.2 to 5.9]	~1.5†† [0 to 3.0]	NR	NR†††
	TURP/ enucleation surgery (n=59)	NR	4.4** (4.9) (n=49)	~4.7† [3.5 to 5.9]	~0.9†† [0 to 2.0]	NR	NR†††
	Mean difference between groups [95% CI]		2.90 [0.46 to 5.34]		NR[a]		
Ghalanyini, 2005[1] RCT 6 months	TURP (n=17)	25.8 (4.2)	-20.3 (8.9)	4.4 (0.9)	-3.0 (1.5)	954 (531)	-854.4 (437)
	CISC (n=24)	23.2 (6.1)	-12.3 (7.8)	4.2 (1.1)	-2.5 (1.4)	963 (503)	-600.5 (537)
	Mean difference between groups [95% CI]		-8.0 [-13.3 to 2.8]		-0.5 [-1.4 to 0.4]		-253.9 [-552.8 to 45.0]
Gujral, 2000 RCT[2] 7.5 months	TURP (n=44)	19.5 (7.2)	-14.2 (8.4) (n=33)	4.5 (2.6) median	-3.2 (1.8) (n=33)	545 (275)	-464 (280) (n=40)
	Laser (n=38)	20.9 (6.4)	-12.2 (9.2) (n=29)	5 (2.6) median	-2.8 (1.7) (n=30)	438 (151)	-329 (135) (n=33)
	Mean difference between groups [95% CI]		-2.0 [-6.4 to 2.4]		-0.4 [-1.3 to 0.5]		-135.0* [-233.2 to -36.8]
	Adj. mean difference between groups [95% CI]		-3.6 [-7.2 to -0.1]		-0.6 [-1.3 to 0.1]		-27.5 [-68.1 to 13]

CI= confidence interval; CISC = clean intermittent self-catheterization; IPSS = International Prostate Symptom Score (range 0 [mild symptoms] to 35 [severe symptoms]; NR = not reported; PLFT = ProstaLund Feedback Treatment; PVR: post-void residual urine volume; QoL = quality of life. IPSS QoL ranges from 1 (delighted) to 6 (terrible); RCT = randomized controlled trial; SD = standard deviation; TURP = transurethral resection of the prostate

[a] could not be calculated.

* Analysis of covariance, adjusting for center effects and baseline measurements, found no statistically significant difference between groups. Difference in means at followup was -27.5 mL [-68.1 to 13.0].

** Mean at endpoint

† Mean score at baseline (extracted from graph)

†† Mean at endpoint (extracted from graph)

††† All patients had PVR volumes over 300 ml at baseline; 2 patients in the TURP group and 4 patients in the TUMT group still had PVR volumes above 300 ml at followup.

Table H4. Comparative effectiveness of treatments for CUR from obstructive causes: adverse events

Study; Design; Followup	Treatment Arms	Death n/N (%)	Septicemia n/N (%)	Blood Transfusion n/N (%)	Major Bleeding n/N (%)	Complication Rate n/N (%)	Serious Adverse Events n/N (%)	Withdrawals
Schelin, 2006[3] RCT 6 months	TUMT (n=61)	NR	NR	NR	NR	NR	1/61 (1.6)	2/61 (3.3)
	TURP/ enucleation surgery (n=59)	NR	NR	NR	NR	NR	5/59 (8.5)	3/59 (5.1)
	Risk ratio [95% CI]						0.19 [0.02 to 1.61]	
Ghalanyini, 2005[1] RCT 6 months	TURP (n=22)	NR	NR	NR	NR	2/17* (11.8)	NR	
	CISC (n=29)	NR	NR	NR	NR	8/24* (33.3)	NR	
	Risk ratio [95% CI]					0.35 [0.09 to 1.46]		
Gujral, 2000 RCT[2] 7.5 months	TURP (n=44)	1/44 (2.3)	3 incidences**	3 incidences**	6 incidences**	13/44 (29.5)	NR	
	Laser (n=38)	0/38 (0.0)	1/38 (2.6)	0/38	0/38	3/38 (7.9)	NR	
	Risk ratio [95% CI]	2.60 [0.11 to 62.01]				3.74 [1.15 to 12.15]		

CI = confidence interval; CISC = clean intermittent self-catheterization; IPSS = International Prostate Symptom Score (range 0 [mild symptoms] to 35 [severe symptoms]); NR = not reported; RCT = randomized controlled trial; TUMT = transurethral microwave therapy; TURP = transurethral resection of the prostate

* Symptomatic infection (6), bleeding (2) or both (2)

** Number of patients unclear

Comparative Effectiveness of Treatments for CUR: Non-Obstructive Causes

Four small efficacy studies and one systematic review compared treatments for CUR attributed to nonobstructive causes in adults. The systematic review was conducted by the Cochrane Incontinence Group and was assessed as being of good quality. Herbison et al. conducted a systematic review evaluating the efficacy of sacral neuromodulation with implanted devices in individuals with voiding dysfunction.[8] They found one RCT that evaluated the efficacy of this intervention in a CUR population. We report the conclusion from that review in lieu of *de novo* abstraction and analysis of the original research addressing that comparison (Table H5).

We identified four studies that compared treatments for CUR attributed to neurogenic disorders in adults. Summary statistics for these studies appear in Table H6. Three of these studies were RCTs with moderate risk of bias, and one was a controlled before-and-after design with a high risk of bias. All four studies were efficacy trials. Studies enrolled a total of 139 patients with sample sizes ranging from 13 to 86. The mean age of enrolled patients was 54 with a range from 46 to 66. Patient sex was fairly evenly distributed with 51 percent men and 49 percent women. Baseline mean IPSS scores were 21.4 across the two studies that measured IPSS, suggesting a severe level of symptoms. Neurogenic disorders among the patients included MS (64 percent), SCI (7 percent), and other (29 percent). Patients had been living with these neurogenic disorders for an average of 13 years in the three studies reporting. Trials were conducted in Europe and Asia. Three studies compared injections of botulinum A into the sphincter to an inactive control (placebo, lidocaine, usual care). The fourth study compared bethanechol/prostaglandin (BC/PGE2) to placebo.

Primary Outcomes

Herbison et al. reviewed sacral neuromodulation with implanted devices for urinary storage and voiding dysfunction in adults.[8] The Cochrane review addressed one comparison relevant to our review, immediate implant versus a delayed implant (i.e., 6-month waitlist control) in treating CUR from nonobstructive retention. We identified one RCT that studied this comparison. At 6 months post-intervention, a greater proportion of the immediate implant group (19/29) no longer needed catheterization compared to the delayed implant group (2/22) with a relative risk of 7.21 [CI: 1.87-27.73]. Those in the immediate implant group also had significantly lower PVR urine volumes. The Cochrane review concludes that sacral neuromodulation with implanted devices is effective in treating nonobstructive CUR. They do not appear to provide strength of evidence for this conclusion.

Only one study reported a primary outcome (Table H7). Gallien, et al. report the rate of UTI at 6 month followup to be 35 percent in the botulinum patients and 29 percent in the placebo patients.[4] This difference was not statistically significant.

Intermediate Outcomes

All four studies reported on at least one of our prespecified intermediate outcomes. (Table H8). Gallien reports IPSS scores at baseline and at 30 day followup for each treatment group. The mean IPSS score improved by three points in the botulinum group, but the placebo group improved by four points.[4] The difference was not significant. In another study of a similar comparison, the botulinum group improved their IPSS mean score by 13 points and the usual care group by only four points.[5] However, this study was not blinded and patients were allowed to select their treatments. Two studies reported quality of life using the IPSS quality of life scale. Hindley et al. found that the botulinum group improved by one point, but the placebo group remained unchanged.[6] Chen et al. found a significant improvement in the botulinum patients over and above the improvement in the usual care patients.[5] Gallien et al., Hindley et al., and de Seze et al. measured PVR at baseline and again at followup. Patients in Gallien et al. had PVRs at baseline of below 300 ml. Both groups showed minimal decreases with no significant difference between groups[4]. Hindley et al. found PVR decreases in both groups from fairly high baseline levels (over 500ml), but only the botulinum patients showed a significant reduction.[6] De Seze et al. also found a significantly greater change in mean PVR in the botulinum group.[7]

Harms

Adverse effects were measured differently in each RCT (Table H9). Adverse effects were rare in all treatment arms. No differences between groups were reported; however, the small sample sizes were likely unable to detect differences in rare events. Strength of evidence was not assessed for harms.

Table H5. Description and conclusions from previous systematic review relevant to treatment for CUR from non-obstructive causes

Study Information	Literature Through; SR Quality	Population; Relevant Comparison	Results; Conclusion Strength of Evidence
Herbison 2009[20] (Cochrane Incontinence Group) Sacral neuromodulation with implanted devices for urinary storage and voiding dysfunction in adults	Literature search through February, 2009 Good	Women with Fowler's syndrome. Immediate/delayed implant (1 trial with CUR patients)	Catheter free: Implant>Delay PVR: Implant>Delay Low

PVR = post void residual; SR=systematic review; UTI = urinary tract infection

Table H6. Comparative effectiveness of treatments for CUR from non-obstructive causes: summary of included studies

Number of studies	4
Randomized controlled trials	3
Number of patients enrolled (range)	139 (13 to 86)
Age of subjects, mean years (range)	54 (46 to 66)
Gender (range)	Men 51% (35 to 92) Women 49% (8 to 65)
Baseline mean IPSS total score (range) (range 0 to 35)*	21.4 (20.5 to 25.0; 2 studies†)
Baseline mean PVR, mL (range)	277 (219 to 530; 3 studies†)
Neurogenic disease etiology	Multiple sclerosis 64% Spinal cord injury 7% Other 29% (stroke, detrusor underactivity)
Neurogenic disease duration, mean years	12.8 (1.4 to 16.1; 3 studies†)
Trials conducted in the United States (% of patients)	None
Trials conducted in Europe (% of patients)	3 (85)
Trials conducted in Asia (% of patients)	1 (15)
Studies reporting primary outcomes	1
Studies reporting secondary outcomes	4

* IPSS = International Prostate Symptom Score: Scoring criteria are: Mild (score 1-7); Moderate (score 8-19); Severe (score 20-35)
† Number of studies reporting this variable

Table H7. Comparative effectiveness of treatments for CUR from non-obstructive causes: primary outcomes

Study; Design; Followup	Treatment Arms	Acute Urinary Retention n/N (%)	Urinary Tract Infection n/N (%)	Catheter Outcomes n/N (%)
Gallien 2005[4] RCT 120 days	botulinum A (n=45)	NR	16/45 (35.6)	NR
	placebo (n=41)	NR	12/41 (29.3)	NR
	RR [95% CI]		1.21 [0.66 to 2.25]	
Hindley 2004[6] RCT 6 weeks	BC/PGE2 (n=9)	NR	NR	NR
	placebo (n=10)	NR	NR	NR
	RR [95% CI]			
De Seze 2002[7] RCT 30 days	botulinum A (n=5)	NR	NR	NR
	lidocaine (n=8)	NR	NR	NR
	RR [95% CI]			
Chen 2004[5] Prospective study 6 months	botulinum A (n=11)	NR	NR	NR
	usual care (n=10)	NR	NR	NR
	RR [95% CI]			

BC/PGE2 = bethanechol chloride/prostaglandin E2; CI = confidence interval; NR = not reported, RR=risk ratio

Table H8. **Comparative effectiveness of treatments for CUR from non-obstructive causes: intermediate outcomes**

Study Design Followup	Treatment Arms	TWOC n/N (%)	IPSS, Mean (SD) Value	Quality of Life Measure	PVR (mL), Mean (SD)
Gallien 2005[4] RCT 30 days	botulinum A (n=43)	NR	Baseline 21 (7)	NR	Baseline 220 (99)
			Endpoint 18 (7)		Endpoint 186 (158)
	placebo (n=40)	NR	Baseline 20 (7)	NR	Baseline 217 (96)
			Endpoint 16 (7)		Endpoint 206 (145)
	Between group comparison ([95% CI] if applicable)		Mean difference at endpoint 2.00 [-1.01 to 5.01]		Mean difference at endpoint -20.00 [-85.19 to 45.19]
Hindley 2004[6] RCT 6 weeks	BC/PGE2 (n=9)	-		Baseline* median (range) 4* (3 to 4.5)	Baseline *median (range)* 426 (405 to 480)
				Endpoint* median (range) 3* (2.5 to 3.5)	Endpoint *median (range)* 325 (290 to 1,252)
	placebo (n=10)			Baseline* median (range) 3.5* (2 to 4)	Baseline *median (range)* 575 (539 to 777)
				Endpoint* median (range) 3.5* (2.5 to 4)	Endpoint *median (range)* 537.5 (350 to 1,775)
	between group comparison ([95% CI] if applicable)			1 point improvement in active arm, unchanged in placebo arm	Significant improvement from baseline in active arm but not placebo arm
de Sèze 2002[7] RCT 30 days	botulinum A (n=5)	NR	NR	NR	Baseline 264.4 (141.3)
					Endpoint 105.0 (100.6)
	lidocaine (n=8)	NR	NR	NR	Baseline 313.1 (138.1)
					Endpoint 263.3 (115.9)
	Between group comparison ([95% CI] if applicable)				Mean difference at endpoint -158.30 [-277.57 to -39.03]
Chen 2004[5] Prospective study 6 months	botulinum A (n=11)	NR	Baseline 27.3 (12.1)	IPSS QoL, baseline 4.7 (1.5)	Baseline 125.5 (88.8)
			Mean change from baseline -13.6 (5.7)	Mean change from baseline 2.4 (1.1)	Endpoint 69.1 (61.4)
	usual care (n=10)	NR	Baseline 22.5 (11.7)	IPSS, baseline 4.3 (2.1)	NR

Study Design Followup	Treatment Arms	TWOC n/N (%)	IPSS, Mean (SD) Value	Quality of Life Measure	PVR (mL), Mean (SD)
			Mean change from baseline -4.1 (5.5)	Mean change from baseline 1.2 (1.0)	
	Between group comparison ([95% CI] if applicable)		Mean difference at endpoint -9.50 [-14.29 to -4.71]	Mean difference at endpoint -1.20 [-2.10 to -0.30]	

BC/ PGE2 = bethanechol chloride/prostaglandin E2; C I= confidence interval; CISC = clean intermittent self-catheterization; IPSS = International Prostate Symptom Score (range 0 [mild symptoms] to 35 [severe symptoms]); NR = not reported; PVR: post-void residual; RCT = randomized controlled trial; RR=risk ratio; SD = standard deviation

* Quality of life scale and range not reported

Table H9. Comparative effectiveness of treatments for CUR from non-obstructive causes: adverse events

Study; Design; Followup	Treatment Arms	Serious Adverse Effects n/N (%)	Urinary Leakage/Incontinence n/N (%)	Any Adverse Event n/N (%)
Gallien, 2005[4] RCT 120 days	botulinum A (n=45)	3/45 (2.2)*	2/45 (4.4)	NR
	placebo (n=41)	3/41 (2.4)*	2/41 (4.9)	NR
	RR [95% CI]	0.91 [0.19 to 4.26]	0.91 [0.13 to 6.18]	
Hindley, 2004[6] RCT 6 weeks	BC/PGE2 (n=9)	0/9 (0.0)	NR	3/9 (33.3)**
	placebo (n=10)	0/10 (0.0)	NR	0/10 (0.0)
	RR [95% CI]	-		7.70 [0.45 to 131.36]
De Seze 2002[7] RCT 30 days	botulinum A (n=5)	0/5 (0.0)	0/5 (20.0)	1/5 (0.0)†
	lidocaine (n=8)	0/8 (12.5)	0/8 (0.0)	1/8 (0.0)†
	RR [95% CI]	-	-	1.60 [0.13 to 20.22]
Chen 2004[5] Prospective study 6 months	botulinum A (n=11)	0/11 (0.0)	NR	NR
	usual care (n=10)	0/10 (0.0)	NR	NR
	RR [95% CI]	-		

BC/ PGE2 = bethanechol chloride/prostaglandin E2; CI = confidence interval; NR = not reported; RR=risk ratio

* Uterine leiomyoma, drug induced confusion, and dyspnoea (one patient in the botulinum A toxin group for each event) and pyelonephritis, lumbar radicular pain, and femoral fracture (one patient in the placebo group for each event)

** Symptomatic adverse effects of BC, including mild lower abdominal cramps, diarrhea and increased perspiration.

† Botulinum - transitory exacerbation of per-existing urine incontinence for 2 weeks, lidocaine -anal incontinence one day after injection

Comparative Effectiveness of CUR Treatments in Adults With Other Causes of CUR

We identified four studies addressing four different comparisons for treatments for CUR from mixed etiologies or etiologies that were not obstructive or neurogenic. One comparison was adequately addressed by a previous systematic reviews. The systematic review was conducted by the Cochrane Incontinence Group. We reviewed the PICOTS and assessed the quality of the review to determine that relevance and quality was sufficient and we identified no new studies comparing the same interventions; therefore, we report conclusions from the relevant systematic review in lieu of *de novo* abstraction and analysis of the original research addressing that comparison.[10] Table H10 summarizes the relevant conclusion from the previous systematic review.

The relevant comparison from the Moore et al. systematic review compared clean versus sterile intermittent catheterization techniques in individuals needing long-term bladder management.[9]

Two RCTs also studied efficacy and comparative effectiveness of CUR interventions in mixed or other populations. Datta et al. conducted a crossover RCT in Europe evaluating the efficacy of sildenafil in women suffering from obstructed voiding or retention associated with Fowler's syndrome.[12] Tang et al. evaluated intermittent versus indwelling catheterization among elderly women with CUR admitted to a geriatric rehabilitation ward.

Primary Outcomes

In assessing the data for clean versus sterile catheterization technique, Moore et al. found the data from three studies insufficient to draw conclusions about the comparative rates of UTI.[9] Only one of these trials was eligible for our review.[10] Because the data from the three trials eligible for the Cochrane review were consistent and this data was assessed insufficient, we reiterate their conclusion of insufficient evidence.

Primary outcomes from the two abstracted studies appear in Table H11. Datta et al. report rates of UTI and successful trial without catheter. Only one patient in either group had a UTI, with no difference between groups.[12] Tang reported only one instance of UTI in either group and TWOC was successful in 59 percent of the intermittent catheter patients and in 69 percent of the indwelling catheter patients.[13] This difference was not statistically significant.

Intermediate Outcomes

Both studies reported several prespecified intermediate outcomes (Table H12). Datta et al. reported before and after data on mean IPSS scores and PVRs. These intermediate outcomes did not improve substantially for either groups and changes from baseline did not differ with statistical significance between sildenafil citrate and placebo patients.[12] Tang et al. report substantial reductions in PVRs after 2 weeks with indwelling versus intermittent catheter; however, the difference was not statistically significant.[13]

Harms

Adverse effects were measured differently in each RCT (Table H13). These events were rare, and results did not differ between treatment groups.

Table H10. Description and conclusions from previous systematic reviews on treatments for CUR in mixed populations/unknown causes

Study Information	Literature Through/SR Quality	Population/Relevant Comparison	Results; Conclusion; Strength of Evidence
Moore, 2007[9] (Cochrane Incontinence Group) Long-term bladder management by intermittent catheterization in adults and children	Literature search through June 2007 Good	Adults and children with incomplete bladder emptying Sterile technique/clean technique (3 trials; only one with only CUR population)	No significant difference in rates of UTI between groups. insufficient
Herbison, 2009[8] (Cochrane Incontinence Group) Sacral neuromodulation with implanted devices for urinary storage and voiding dysfunction in adults	Literature search through February 2009 Good	Women with Fowler's syndrome. Immediate/delayed implant (1 trial with CUR patients)	Catheter free: Implant>Delay PVR: Implant>Delay Strength of evidence – not reported; Author's conclude 'Continuous stimulation offers benefits for urinary retention without obstruction.'

UTI = urinary tract infection; PVR = post void residual urine volume

Table H11. Comparative effectiveness of treatments for CUR in mixed populations/unknown causes: primary outcomes

Study; Design; Followup	Treatment Arms	Acute Urinary Retention n/N (%)	Urinary Tract Infection n/N (%)	Surgical Intervention n/N (%)	IPSS n/N (%)	TWOC n/N (%)
Datta, 2007[12] Randomized crossover trial 10 weeks	sildenafil citrate (n=20)	NR	1/20 (0.05)	NR	NR	NR
Tang, 2006[13] RCT 2 weeks	placebo (n=20)	NR	0/20 (0.0) No statistically significant difference	NR	NR	NR
	RR [95% CI]					
	RR [95% CI]		3.73 [0.16 to 88.90]			0.86 [0.59 to 1.25]

CI = confidence interval; IDC = indwelling urinary catheterization; IMC = intermittent urinary catheterization; IPSS = International Prostate Symptom Score (range 0 [mild symptoms] to 35 [severe symptoms]; NR = not reported; RCT = randomized controlled trial; TWOC = successful trial without catheter

Table H12. Comparative effectiveness of treatments for CUR in mixed populations/unknown causes: intermediate outcomes

Study; Design; Followup	Treatment Arms	IPSS, Mean (SD) Value	Quality of Life Measure	PVR (mL), Mean (SD)
Datta, 2007[12] Randomized crossover trial 10 weeks	sildenafil citrate (n=20)	Baseline 21.5* [20 to 23]	NR	Baseline 140* [90 to 180]
		Mean change from baseline -3.6		Endpoint 90* [70 to 120]
	placebo (n=20)	Baseline 21.5* [20 to 23]	NR	Baseline 140* [90 to 180]
		Endpoint 19* [18 to 20]		Endpoint 99* [70 to 130]
	Between group comparison ([95% CI] if applicable)	Mean difference at endpoint. No statistically significant difference		Mean difference at endpoint: no statistically significant difference
Tang, 2006[13] RCT 2 weeks	IMC (n=27)	NR	NR	Baseline 539.8 (219.7)
				Endpoint 54.4 (49.1)
	IDC (n=39)	NR	NR	Baseline 545.9 (187.2)
				Endpoint 77.6 (48.2)
	Between group comparison ([95% CI] if applicable)			Mean difference at endpoint -23.20 [-47.03 to 0.63]

IDC = indwelling urinary catheterization; IMC = intermittent urinary catheterization; NR = no response; SD = standard deviation

* Extracted from graph

Table H13. Comparative effectiveness of treatments for CUR in mixed populations/unknown causes: adverse events

Study; Design; Followup	Treatment Arms	Death n/N (%)	Clinical Deterioration n/N (%)	Urinary Leakage/ Incontinence n/N (%)	Total Adverse Events n/N (%)
Datta, 2007[12] Randomized crossover trial 10 weeks	sildenafil citrate (n=20)	0/20 (0.0)	NR	0/20 (0.0)	14/20 (0.7)
	Placebo (n=20)	1/20 (0.05)	NR	1/20 (0.05)	14/20 (0.7)
	RR [95% CI]	No statistically significant difference		No statistically significant difference	No statistically significant difference
Tang, 2006[13] RCT 2 weeks	IMC (n=36)	0/36 (0.0)	4/36 (11.1)	NR	NR
	IDC (n=45)	2/45 (4.4)	1/45 (2.2)	NR	NR
	RR [95% CI]	0.25 [0.01 to 5.02]	5.00 [0.58 to 42.80]		

IDC = indwelling urinary catheterization; IMC = intermittent urinary catheterization; NR = not reported; RR=risk ratio

* Based on number of urine cultures sent on day 14.

References for Appendix H

1. Ghalayini IF, Al-Ghazo MA, Pickard RS. A prospective randomized trial comparing transurethral prostatic resection and clean intermittent self-catheterization in men with chronic urinary retention. BJU International. 2005 Jul;96(1):93-7. PMID 15963128.
2. Gujral S, Abrams P, Donovan JL, et al. A prospective randomized trial comparing transurethral resection of the prostate and laser therapy in men with chronic urinary retention: The CLasP study. Journal of Urology. 2000 Jul;164(1):59-64. PMID 10840425.
3. Schelin S, Geertsen U, Walter S, et al. Feedback microwave thermotherapy versus TURP/prostate enucleation surgery in patients with benign prostatic hyperplasia and persistent urinary retention: a prospective, randomized, controlled, multicenter study. Urology. 2006 Oct;68(4):795-9. PMID 17070355.
4. Gallien P, Reymann JM, Amarenco G, et al. Placebo controlled, randomised, double blind study of the effects of botulinum A toxin on detrusor sphincter dyssynergia in multiple sclerosis patients. Journal of Neurology, Neurosurgery & Psychiatry. 2005 Dec;76(12):1670-6. PMID 16291892.
5. Chen YH, Kuo HC. Botulinum A toxin treatment of urethral sphincter pseudodyssynergia in patients with cerebrovascular accidents or intracranial lesions. Urologia Internationalis. 2004;73(2):156-61; discussion 61-2. PMID 15331901.
6. Hindley RG, Brierly RD, Thomas PJ. Prostaglandin E2 and bethanechol in combination for treating detrusor underactivity. BJU International. 2004 Jan;93(1):89-92. PMID 14678375.
7. de Seze M, Petit H, Gallien P, et al. Botulinum a toxin and detrusor sphincter dyssynergia: a double-blind lidocaine-controlled study in 13 patients with spinal cord disease. European Urology. 2002 Jul;42(1):56-62. PMID 12121731.
8. Herbison GP, Arnold EP. Sacral neuromodulation with implanted devices for urinary storage and voiding dysfunction in adults. Cochrane Database of Systematic Reviews. 2009(2):CD004202. PMID 19370596.
9. Moore K, N., Fader M, Getliffe K. Long-term bladder management by intermittent catheterisation in adults and children. John Wiley & Sons, Ltd; 2007. http://onlinelibrary.wiley.com/doi/10.1002/14651858.CD006008.pub2/abstract. Accessed on 4.
10. Duffy LM, Cleary J, Ahern S, et al. Clean intermittent catheterization: safe, cost-effective bladder management for male residents of VA nursing homes. Journal of the American Geriatrics Society. 1995 Aug;43(8):865-70. PMID 7636093.
11. Jonas U, Fowler CJ, Chancellor MB, et al. Efficacy of sacral nerve stimulation for urinary retention: results 18 months after implantation. Journal of Urology. 2001 Jan;165(1):15-9. PMID 11125353.
12. Datta SN, Kavia RB, Gonzales G, et al. Results of double-blind placebo-controlled crossover study of sildenafil citrate (Viagra) in women suffering from obstructed voiding or retention associated with the primary disorder of sphincter relaxation (Fowler's Syndrome). European Urology. 2007 Feb;51(2):489-95; discussion 95-7. PMID 16884844.
13. Tang MW, Kwok TC, Hui E, et al. Intermittent versus indwelling urinary catheterization in older female patients. Maturitas. 2006 Feb 20;53(3):274-81. PMID 16084677.

Appendix I. Strength of Evidence

Appendix Table I1. Strength of evidence assessments: comparative effectiveness of treatments for CUR from obstructive causes

Comparison; # of Studies; N	Outcomes	Summary Statistics [95% CI]	Risk of Bias	Directness	Precision	Consistency	Evidence Rating
Microwave therapy vs. TURP or prostate enucleation surgery	**Primary Outcomes**						
	Urinary tract infection	RR 1.49 [95% CI 0.82 to 2.71]	Moderate	Direct	Imprecise	Single study	Insufficient
	Catheter-free status	RR 0.89 [95% CI 0.76 to 1.05]	Moderate	Direct	Precise	Single study	Low
	Intermediate Outcomes						
1 RCT	IPSS, mean at endpoint	MD 2.9 [95%CI 0.5 to 5.3]	Moderate	Indirect	Imprecise	Single study	Insufficient
	IPSS QoL, mean change	NS between interventions*	Moderate	Indirect	Unclear	Single study	Insufficient
N=120	PVR (ml)	Not reported	-	-	-	-	Insufficient
TURP vs. clean intermittent self-catheterization	**Primary Outcomes**						
	None reported		-	-	-	-	
	Intermediate Outcomes						
1 RCT	IPSS, mean at endpoint	MD -8.0 [95%CI -13.3 to 2.8]	Moderate	Indirect	Imprecise	Single study	Insufficient
	IPSS QoL, mean change	MD -0.5 [95%CI -1.4 to 0.4]	Moderate	Indirect	Imprecise	Single study	Insufficient
N=51	PVR (ml)	MD -254 [95%CI -553 to 45]	Moderate	Indirect	Imprecise	Single study	Insufficient
TURP vs. laser therapy	**Primary Outcomes**						
	Urinary tract infection	RR 1.73 [95% CI 0.16 to 18.31]	High	Direct	Imprecise	Single study	Insufficient
1 RCT	IPSS category, adjusted	RR 1.27 [95% CI 0.97 to 1.68]	Moderate	Direct	Imprecise	Single study	Insufficient
	Intermediate Outcomes						
	IPSS, mean at endpoint	MD -2.0 [95%CI -6.4 to 2.4]	Moderate	Indirect	Imprecise	Single study	Insufficient
N=82	IPSS QoL, mean change	MD -0.4 [95%CI -1.3 to 0.5]	Moderate	Indirect	Imprecise	Single study	Insufficient
	PVR (ml), adjusted	MD -135 [95%CI -233 to -37]	Moderate	Indirect	Precise	Single study	Low

RR = relative risk [95 percent confidence intervals]; MD = mean difference [95 percent confidence intervals]; TURP = transurethral resection of the prostate; NS = No statistically significant difference.

* Mean difference could not be calculated

Table I2. Strength of evidence assessments: comparative effectiveness of treatments for CUR from non-obstructive causes

Study; Comparison; N	Outcomes	Summary Statistics [95% CI]	Risk of Bias	Directness	Precision	Consistency	Evidence Rating
Botulinum A toxin injected into sphincter vs. placebo 1 RCT N=86	**Primary Outcomes**						
	Urinary tract infection	RR 1.21 [95% CI 0.66 to 2.25]	Moderate	Direct	Imprecise	Single study	Insufficient
	Intermediate Outcomes						
	IPSS, mean at endpoint	MD 2.0 [95%CI -1.0 to 5.0]	Moderate	Indirect	Imprecise	Single study	Insufficient
	IPSS QoL, mean change	Not reported	-	-	-	-	Insufficient
	PVR (ml)	MD -20 [95%CI -85 to 45]	Moderate	Indirect	Imprecise	Single study	Insufficient
Bethanechol chloride plus prostaglandin E2 vs. placebo 1 RCT N=19	**Primary Outcomes**						
	Urinary tract infection	Not reported	-	-	-	-	Insufficient
	Intermediate Outcomes						
	IPSS, mean at endpoint	Not reported	-	-	-	-	Insufficient
	QoL, mean change	NS between interventions*	High	Indirect	Imprecise	Single study	Insufficient
	PVR (ml)	NS between interventions*	Moderate	Indirect	Imprecise	Single study	Insufficient
Botulinum A toxin injected into sphincter vs. Lidocaine 1 RCT N=13	**Primary Outcomes**						
	Urinary tract infection	Not reported	-	-	-	-	Insufficient
	Intermediate Outcomes						
	IPSS, mean at endpoint	Not reported	-	-	-	-	Insufficient
	IPSS QoL, mean change	Not reported	-	-	-	-	Insufficient
	PVR (ml)	MD 538 [95% CI 350 to 1775]	Moderate	Indirect	Imprecise	Single study	Insufficient
Botulinum A toxin injected into sphincter vs. Lidocaine 1 Prospective study	**Primary Outcomes**						
	Urinary tract infection	Not reported	-	-	-	-	Insufficient
	Intermediate Outcomes						
	IPSS, mean at endpoint	MD -9.5 [95%CI -14.3 to -4.7]	High	Indirect	Imprecise	Single study	Insufficient
	IPSS QoL, mean change	MD -1.2 [95%CI -2.1 to -0.3]	High	Indirect	Imprecise	Single study	Insufficient
	PVR (ml)	MD -135 [95%CI -233 to -37]	High	Indirect	Imprecise	Single study	Insufficient
Sacral neuromodulation with implanted device: Immediate vs. delayed implant SR N=21	**Primary Outcomes**						
	Catheter free	RR 7.21 [95% CI 1.87 to 27.73]	SR: Low	Direct	Precise	Single study	Low
	Intermediate Outcomes						
	PVR (ml)	MD -1068 [95% CI -1493 to -643]	Moderate	Indirect	Precise	Single study	Low

SR=systematic review; RR = relative risk [95 percent confidence intervals] MD = mean difference [95 percent confidence intervals]; NS = No statistically significant difference.

* Mean difference could not be calculated

Appendix Table I3. Strength of evidence assessments: comparative effectiveness of treatments for CUR: mixed populations/unknown causes

Study; Comparison; N	Outcomes	Summary Statistics [95% CI]	Risk of Bias	Directness	Precision	Consistency	Evidence Rating
Sildenafil vs. placebo 1 RCT N=19	**Primary Outcomes**						
	Acute urinary retention	Not reported	-	-	-	-	Insufficient
	Urinary tract infection	1 event in sildenafil arm	Moderate	Direct	Imprecise	Single study	Insufficient
	Surgical intervention	Not reported	-	-	-	-	Insufficient
	Treatment failure	Not reported	-	-	-	-	Insufficient
	Catheter outcomes	Not reported	-	-	-	-	Insufficient
	Intermediate Outcomes						
	IPSS, mean at endpoint	NS between interventions*	Moderate	Indirect	Imprecise	Single study	Insufficient
	QoL, mean change	Not reported	-	-	-	-	Insufficient
	PVR (ml)	NS between interventions*	Moderate	Indirect	Imprecise	Single study	Insufficient
Intermittent urinary catheterization vs. indwelling urinary catheterization 1 RCT N=81	**Primary Outcomes**						
	Acute urinary retention	Not reported	-	-	-	-	Insufficient
	Urinary tract infection	1 event in IMC arm	Moderate	Direct	Imprecise	Single study	Insufficient
	Surgical intervention	Not reported	-	-	-	-	Insufficient
	Treatment failure	Not reported	-	-	-	-	Insufficient
	Catheter outcomes	RR 0.86 [95% CI 0.59 to 1.25]	Moderate	Direct	Imprecise	Single study	Insufficient
	Intermediate Outcomes						
	IPSS, mean at endpoint	Not reported	-	-	-	-	Insufficient
	QoL, mean change	Not reported	-	-	-	-	Insufficient
	PVR (ml)	MD -23 [95% CI -47 to 0.63]	Moderate	Indirect	Precise	Single study	Low

Single study = not applicable; RR = relative risk [95 percent confidence intervals]; MD = mean difference [95 percent confidence intervals]; NS = No statistically significant difference.

* Mean difference could not be calculated

Appendix J. Ongoing Studies

Table J1. Ongoing studies

NCT Number	Title	Conditions	Interventions	Study Designs
NCT01460303	Patient-operated Valved Catheter Versus Indwelling Transurethral Catheter	Bladder Dysfunction|Urinary Retention	Device: Bladder catheter: OPTION-vf patient controlled catheter vs. indwelling transurethral catheter with leg bag Device: Transurethral catheter with leg bag	Allocation: Randomized|Endpoint Classification: Efficacy Study|Intervention Model: Parallel Assignment|Masking: Open Label|Primary Purpose: Treatment
NCT00878176	Sacral Neuromodulation Test With Bilateral First Stage Tined Lead Procedure in Patients with Non-obstructive Urinary Retention: A Pilot Study	Urinary Retention	Procedure: First stage tined lead procedure	Endpoint Classification: Efficacy Study|Intervention Model: Crossover Assignment|Masking: Open Label|Primary Purpose: Screening
NCT00680680	Treatment of Refractory Urinary Retention Secondary to Benign Prostatic Hyperplasia (BPH) with Dual Five Alpha Reductase Inhibition Combined with an Alpha Blocker	Urinary Retention|Benign Prostatic Hyperplasia	Drug: Dutasteride	Allocation: Non-Randomized|Endpoint Classification: Efficacy Study|Intervention Model: Single Group Assignment|Masking: Open Label|Primary Purpose: Treatment
NCT00700505	A Study to Determine the Safety and Efficacy of a New Non-invasive Heating Garment to Reduce Urinary Hesitancy	Benign Prostatic Hyperplasia (BPH)|Urinary Retention|Urinary Hesitancy Intermittent	Device: FlowPants(R) Garment	Endpoint Classification: Safety/Efficacy Study|Intervention Model: Single Group Assignment|Masking: Open Label|Primary Purpose: Treatment
NCT00441935	InterStim Prospective Database	Urinary Retention|Urinary Incontinence|Pelvic Pain	Device: InterStim Neuromodulation	Time Perspective: Prospective
NCT00970242	Ambulatory Urodynamic Evaluation of Sacral Neuromodulation for Non-Obstructive Urinary Retention	Acontractile Bladder		Time Perspective: Prospective
NCT01404481	Clean Intermittant Self Catheterisation: A Trial Comparing Single Use vs. Reuse of Nelaton Catheters	Urinary Retention	Device: clean intermittent self catheterisation single use vs. re use	Observational Model: Cohort|Time Perspective: Prospective
NCT01771159	Tissue Bonding Cystostomy (TBC)	Spinal Cord Injury (SCI)|Chronic Urinary Retention|Urinary Incontinence	Device: TBC	Intervention Model: Single Group Assignment|Masking: Open Label|Primary Purpose: Treatment

NCT Number	Title	Conditions	Interventions	Study Designs
NCT01164280	Effect of Pulse Rate Changes on Clinical Outcome	Overactive Bladder Syndrome|Chronic Urinary Retention	Other: Pulse Rate Change	Intervention Model: Single Group Assignment|Primary Purpose: Treatment
NCT00883220	Self Management in Urinary Catheter Users	Urinary Retention|Neurogenic Bladder	Behavioral: Self-management of urinary catheter	Allocation: Randomized|Endpoint Classification: Safety/Efficacy Study|Intervention Model: Parallel Assignment|Masking: Single Blind (Investigator)|Primary Purpose: Prevention
NCT00225966	Patient Registry to Study the Tined Lead Used with the InterStim System for Urinary Control	Urge Incontinence|Urinary Retention	Device: Device Medtronic InterStim Tined Leads Models 3889 and 3093	Allocation: Non-Randomized|Endpoint Classification: Safety/Efficacy Study|Intervention Model: Single Group Assignment|Masking: Open Label|Primary Purpose: Treatment
NCT01284361	Comparison of Two Intermittent Urinary Catheters	Urinary Retention	Device: test and control intermittent urinary catheters	Allocation: Randomized|Intervention Model: Crossover Assignment|Masking: Open Label
NCT01305681	Bacterial Properties with LoFric® Catheters During Clean Intermittent Catheterization	Neurogenic Bladder|Urinary Retention	Device: LoFric® catheters during clean intermittent catheterization	Allocation: Non-Randomized|Intervention Model: Parallel Assignment|Masking: Open Label|Primary Purpose: Treatment
NCT00200031	A Cost Analysis of Interstim Therapy	Urinary Retention and Symptoms of Overactive Bladder (Urge, Frequency)	Device: Interstim therapy	
NCT01130415	Screening Method in Sacral Neuromodulation	Overactive Bladder|Urinary Retention		Observational Model: Cohort|Time Perspective: Retrospective

Appendix K. Future Research Needs

Table K1. Future research needs

Key Question	Results of Literature Review	Types of Studies Needed To Answer Question	Future Research Recommendations
General	Many of the studies on interventions for CUR were uncontrolled Intervention studies enrolling men with CUR and BPH typically also required them to have significant lower urinary tract symptoms, not possible to differentiate whether improvements reflect the treatment for CUR or LUTS when they have overlapping interventions Intervention studies enrolling neurogenic bladder patients rarely described type of voiding dysfunction	Observational Qualitative Consensus development	Research to describe the natural history of CUR Standardized definition of CUR Clearly separate AUR and CUR patients in research studies Studies that evaluate if, when, and who it is beneficial to screen for CUR Make determination whether CUR should be addressed as a separate condition or better addressed as a manifestation of the underlying condition Design intervention studies in the neurogenic bladder population that include adequate numbers of different types of neurogenic bladder (incontinent, retention, both) to determine if outcomes vary by type of voiding dysfunction Conduct controlled studies on CUR interventions Studies with adequately powered subgroups of CUR patients should be conducted to determine whether CUR modifies the effect of treatment Only conduct studies that are adequately powered
1a. What is the effectiveness and comparative effectiveness of treatments for chronic urinary retention in adults, male-specific etiologies?	Only three trials were identified. No two studies compared the same interventions BPH was the only male-specific etiology studied We identified no studies that examined BPH as a subgroup of a larger trial Data was identified for only four interventions No data for long-term outcomes available	RCTs; prospective cohort studies	Additional studies necessary to establish consistency for TURP Efficacy and comparative effectiveness of pharmaceutical interventions such as alpha blockers and 5 alpha reductase inhibitors[a] Studies with followup times extending for several years

Key Question	Results of Literature Review	Types of Studies; Needed To Answer Question	Future Research Recommendations
1b. What is the effectiveness and comparative effectiveness of treatments for chronic urinary retention in adults, female-specific etiologies?	Only one study addressed a predominantly female etiology (Fowler's syndrome) Only one patient-centered outcome was evaluated No data for long-term outcomes available	RCTs; prospective cohort studies	Controlled studies of interventions for women with CUR resulting from SUI procedures or from pelvic organ prolapse Intervention studies with nonimplanted devices to treat Fowler's syndrome Controlled studies of neuromodulation interventions with long-term followup to determine duration of effectiveness
1c. What is the effectiveness and comparative effectiveness of treatments for chronic urinary retention in adults, nonsex-specific etiologies?	We identified few studies that addressed nonsex-specific etiologies Neurogenic bladder was the only etiology studied Studies often enrolled populations with heterogeneous underlying conditions Small sample sizes Primarily intermediate outcomes studied	RCTs, prospective cohort studies	Additional patient-centered outcomes should be included
1d. What patient or condition characteristics (e.g., age, severity, etc.) modify the effectiveness of treatment?	One study used a more conservative treatment in men with higher prostate volumes	RCTs, prospective cohort studies	Stratify enrolled CUR patients by severity
2a. What are the harms and comparative harms of treatments for chronic urinary retention in adults with male-specific, female-specific, and nonsex-specific etiologies?	Harms were inconsistently measured and reported		Adequately collect and report data on harms.
2d. What patient or condition characteristics (e.g., age, severity, etc.) modify the harms of treatment?	Not addressed by current literature		Larger sample sizes will enable this type of analysis

[a] One RCT was identified in Clinicaltrials.gov; completed in 2008, but results are not available

www.ingramcontent.com/pod-product-compliance
Lightning Source LLC
Chambersburg PA
CBHW081736170526
45167CB00009B/3842